FOLLOWING THE DOCTOR'S ORDERS

My resident instructed me to place an intravenous line and write my admitting orders. Later, we would reconnoiter and decide on a further plan of action.

I stuck the IV into Mr. Kram's tissuelike veins and traipsed off to write his orders. They would contain such helpful and useful instructions as "activities: bed rest with bathroom privileges," and "diet: low salt/kosher." When I was finished, I wandered off to attack another patient, some poor soul whose IV had come out, was leaking, hurting, or whatever. As an intern I spent more time messing about with IVs than monks do meditating.

While prodding the next patient, I suddenly realized that I'd left Mr. Kram's IV wide open, allowing fluid to pour unrestrained into him. I zipped down the hall and up the stairs to his room and stopped dead on arriving at his bedside. The IV bag hung completely empty above the patient, who was sitting up in bed with his legs crossed and his face hidden by a newspaper.

Mr. Kram, apparently, had been a bit dry. That was the last time I had any fun with him.

MORPHINE, ICE CREAM TEARS

Tales of a City Hospital

Joseph Sacco, M.D.

PINNACLE BOOKS
WINDSOR PUBLISHING CORP.

PINNACLE BOOKS

are published by

Windsor Publishing Corp.
475 Park Avenue South
New York, NY 10016

First Pinnacle Books printing: November, 1990

Printed in the United States of America

For my parents

Contents

1

Nighttime at the Cloud Pavilion

I was on call one night at the Cloud Pavilion, running around at four in the morning tormenting elderly people. I had a new patient, a man who must have been tremendous when he was younger, like a football player or a sumo wrestler, because at the age of eighty he was still gigantic. I remember being impressed by his size and somewhere, dimly, feeling sadness that illness had reduced him to a helpless, dying, mindless shell of what he had once been.

The old fellow lay in a bed in one of the private rooms. I could hear him coughing up a ruckus from down the corridor, oblivious to the nightmare of "medical care" that would shortly lay waste his body and dignity. I walked to his room and stopped at the door to gaze in at him. He continued to cough, spewing spittle and bacteria into the stagnant hospital air.

I was the patient's intern, a job I'd begun only weeks before, at the age of twenty-six, when I'd been flung headlong from the status and safety of the senior year of medical school into the maw of modern American in-hospital training. These few weeks had transformed me into a haggard, sleepless, disheveled hospital workhorse. School, and any bright-eyed eagerness that may have accompanied it, lay a thousand years in my past; the end of internship, still almost a year of 80- to 120-hour work weeks ahead, a thousand years in my future.

For absolutely no reason at all, I named my new charge

Uncle Melvin. As his intern my job was to "treat" him to provide him with appropriate, well-reasoned, and well-planned medical care. Like a child torturing a hapless slug on a beach, I would torment him relentlessly, poking, prodding, irradiating, poisoning, and sticking him with every imaginable gauge of needle until he was cured, transferred, or dead.

The patient had been delivered into my hands for invasion and treatment regardless of the fact that he had long since lost the capacity to understand, never mind consent to, his "management" in the hospital. I suspected that somewhere deep in his brain were the gatherings, the essence, primitive, possibly merely visceral, of a refusal to consent to what would happen next.

I proceeded into his room. I didn't care, at 4:00 A.M., what or if Uncle Melvin thought. My immediate problem was purely practical. The patient had pneumonia and as intern I was obligated to do the "scut," the work, the "work-up" on him; medical history, physical examination, blood tests, X rays, orders, and on and on and on, ad infinitum, ad nauseam.

Because he suffered a "dense dementia," what might popularly be called senility, and had not uttered a sentence in years, a coherent sentence in decades, I was saved the time-consuming task of taking his "history," an interview regarding the patient's physical complaints and past medical problems. Instead, I would refer to the "Nursing Home Transfer Summary," a sheet of paper that had accompanied him when he was consigned to Cloud from the nursing home that was his usual site of incarceration.

This form, a tenuous, jargon-packed summary of the patient's medical misadventures, read, "Past Medical History: status-post pneumonia x4, status-post urinary tract infection x3, status-post multiple CVAs, dense dementia, colon cancer, stage 4 decubitus on right buttock." A catastrophic litany, this list told me most of all that the patient was a cornucopia of chronic, debilitating disease. "Status-post" was medical lingo meaning that a given condition had occurred in the past. Uncle Melvin had already suffered several infections in his lungs and pee-pee (the urinary tract), each of which, undoubtedly, had required hospitalization. "CVA" was shorthand for "cerebrovascular accident," or, simply, stroke. That the old fellow had "multiple" CVAs signified that he'd had more strokes than anyone could, or bothered to, remember. Other of his problems were ongoing, like cancer of the large intestine (colon) and a senility so severe his IQ could be guessed by rolling a pair of dice. "Stage 4 decubitus on right buttock" indicated that he'd spent so many years lying in bed that he had a bed sore reaching right down to the bone.

Under "Primary Diagnosis," that portion of the form meant to detail the reason the man had been sent to the hospital on this particular day, I would find inscribed a medical condition related only randomly to what the patient might actually have. Melvin, whose pneumonia was obvious from the end of the hall, was advertised as "rule-out GI [gastrointestinal] bleed."

"Ruling out" a condition, establishing that it did not exist in a patient, was a common cause for admission. We might, for example, admit a man with chest pain to make sure that he was not having a heart attack, rather than risk his dropping dead at home. If in-hospital testing determined that the heart was not the cause of the pain, the patient might then be safely discharged. In all likelihood the doc or nurse at the nursing home, in an absolute panic to dump Uncle Melvin, decided that "rule-out GI bleed" was an ideal way to dupe the hospital into admitting a patient with colon cancer, a potentially bleeding tumor in his intestines. Pneumonia might legitimately be managed in the nursing home; "rule-out GI bleed," however, threatened that the patient might bleed to death into his guts and assured a successful "turf" to the hospital. In my opinion, it was the doc or nurse who filled out the form that needed admission. We'd work 'em right up the wazoo for "rule-out total stupidity."

In fact, Melvin's "Nursing Home Transfer Summary" sheet was about par, about average when compared to those of my other nursing home patients. It was worthless.

That Melvin himself was incapable of giving a history made my job much easier. When detailing his history in his hospital chart I would merely quote, verbatim, the inept transfer sheet and add, "Patient unable to give further history."

Despite such welcome simplicity in dealing with this aspect of his case, I would still have to examine him, and subject his snot, urine, blood, and virtually any other body fluid obtainable with a needle or plastic tube to scrutiny in the lab. Holding my breath, I would still have to descend into the bowels of the hospital to the Kafkaesque X-ray file room and beg, teary-eyed, with its staff to locate and release to me Uncle Melvin's chest X ray.

I was certain to fail. The X-ray file room was actually created to ensure that interns never, *ever*, locate their patients' X rays. Yet, like a doughboy saber charging a machine-gun nest, I would face the task despite insurmountable odds; these were my orders.

Next, I would discuss Melvin's in-hospital management with my supervising resident. By virtue of surviving the internship year, this poor slob had graduated from inmate to trustee, slave to gang leader, at the same time I'd been demoted from medical student to intern just those few endless weeks earlier. Together we would agree on a formidable array of nephro(kidney)toxic, oto(ear)toxic, neuro(nerve) toxic, and hepato(liver)toxic antibiotics, biochemical mutants, to ice Uncle Melvin's pneumonia and possibly ice Uncle Melvin, too.

We would write separate notes in his chart and I'd write his admitting orders. This completed, Melvin ("Melvin, Uncle") would become an official patient on the Cloud Pavilion at Manhattan Hospital, considered by many to be New York City's finest private medical institution, and known fondly to its staff as "MH."

Uncle Melvin had pneumonia but not enough brain

function to understand the need to cough up a glob of phlegm for me to play with in the lab. Phlegm, layered out on a slide, stained with red and blue dye, and scrutinized under the microscope for bugs, is the centerpiece, the crowning event, the pièce de résistance of the pneumonia work-up. It was imperative for me to get some.

Since he would not, indeed could not, cough some up for me, I would have to hold him down and use a snorting, sucking flexible plastic tube to forcibly take some. I'd shove the tube into his nose, push it right down next to his wind-pipe (trachea), and use the suction apparatus attached to the wall in his room to draw it up, thickly veined with blood and pus, right from the seething heart of the pneumonia. After taking the sample of snot to the lab, I'd tease it onto a microscope slide with a cotton swab and, peering at a seg-ment enlarged in such a way that the entire sample equally magnified would engulf the whole Cloud Pavilion, I would retch but not quite lose my cookies.

I tried reasoning with the patient.

"Melvin," I said, "I'm going to ram this tube down your nose. I'm going to do so whether you like it or not."

I paused, scrutinizing his impassive face for the slightest flicker of understanding. Lizardlike, he gazed back at me.

"Now, Melvin," I continued, shaking the sucking tube for emphasis. "It's going to be easier and faster for both of us if you lie still while I do this."

At this moment the scene in Uncle Melvin's room on Cloud 3 exceeded any reasonable definition of normalcy. Here, a normal individual, someone with a normal job, a normal family, a normal life, might rationally consider him-self witness to a tableau combining elements of Salvador Dali, Franz Kafka, Edvard Munch, and Dachau. Sprawled haphazardly in a hospital bed lies the large bulk of a man somewhere between 75 and 120 years of age, the spittle dribbling down his chin clearly indicative of well-progressed senescence. Seated on the bed next to the gentleman is an intern, a young man in his mid-twenties, his white pants and white lab jacket splotched with coagulated blood and

13

other, less identifiable, human fluids and excreta. The intern, a product of eight years of postsecondary education, waves a strange, snorting, clear plastic tube menacingly before the old man's face. For a few moments he appears to be pleading with his victim in incoherent, near inaudible, babbling tones. Suddenly, he plunges the tube into the man's nose.

I plunged the tube into Uncle Melvin's nose.

In keeping with my burgeoning roster of combat experiences with demented patients, he began to struggle immediately. I'd discovered that no matter how gorked out the patient, he will still fight when hurt. Perhaps the part of the brain responsible for responding to pain is the oldest, the last to go after the rest has slowly wasted away. Even the primitive, hapless, tortured sea slug withdraws when prodded by the gleeful child. Melvin, in the most human of the interactions we'd had as yet, grunted and pushed at my hand as I tried to shove the tube farther into his nose.

I paused. There is a maxim in medicine that there is no body cavity or fluid an intern cannot reach given the appropriate gauge needle (or the right size tube) and a strong right arm. The pus in Melvin's lungs would prove no exception to this rule despite his lack of cooperation or consent. I would simply tie him down to the bed and "snake" him again. "Snaking" was the intern's phrase for the process of invading a patient with a sucking tube in order to extract snot.

I snatched a few rolls of stretchable bandage from the supply closet at the nurses' station and set to work securing Melvin's sumo wrestler body onto the bed. Soon, his arms, legs, and trunk were tightly fastened. Only his head helplessly lolled about. I would now firmly hold his head with one hand while mercilessly, relentlessly passing the tube with the other.

I hesitated before beginning. Melvin seemed quite content. Like the persecuted slug, he'd forgotten the torture as soon as the noxious stimulus ceased. He was back somewhere in a vacant timeless place I knew nothing of. Perhaps

14

he was cradling the first of his newborn children or in a passioned embrace with the first of his loves. Maybe he was in the womb.

I used the tube to bring him back to the present, and the shrieking and grunting resumed. His head, despite considerable restraining pressure, still managed to flail about. I imagined that he must have had a hell of a head punch back in his sumo wrestler days. I began to sweat the sixth or seventh layer of sweat I had shed in the preceding twenty or so hours. In the next fifteen or sixteen hours I would sweat a good eight or ten layers more. Each would capture and lock next to my body the particular odor, be it shit, piss, or vomit, characterizing the location in which I was sweating, along with the all-pervasive, sharp smell of ammonia-based disinfectant.

The total of thirty-four to forty hours straight I'd spend in the hospital, only a fraction of which would be necessary to complete the torture of Uncle Melvin, comprised being "on call," the essence of the intern's experience. A typical day on call began anywhere from six to eight in the morning and progressed nonstop until the night of the following day. By forcing docs in training to work such catastrophically long hours, the hospital managed to provide twenty-four-hour medical coverage with a minimum of staff. All of the other hospital personnel worked in normal shifts. Nurses, for example, had a "day shift" from 7:00 A.M. to 3:00 P.M., an "evening shift" from 3:00 to 11:00 P.M., and a "night shift" from 11:00 P.M. to 7:00 A.M. The docs had no set hours. While the nurses worked a 40-hour week, the interns and residents, members of the "housestaff," worked 80 to 120 hours per week. An intern's pay, broken down to an hourly rate, was under minimum wage.

While on call, an intern admits new patients to the hospital, either those sent by private doctors or people from the emergency room, and does the nitty-gritty of patient care. These tasks include an endless grind of paperwork, three to four hours daily of telephone calls, sticking sick people with needles, chasing down lab results and X rays, and so on, very little of which contributes to the actual welfare of the patients.

Although the responsibility to admit new patients ends early in the morning after a night on call, the intern's duty to attend both old and new patients continues. Sleep-deprived and haggard, he spends the next day slogging through a "scut list" of tasks—blood tests for Mr. Jones, X rays for Mrs. Smith, snot results for Uncle Melvin, and so on—until the day's work is done. The intern has no contract, no set hours or stopping time, and leaves when the work is finished. In general, the longer he stays, the more work presents itself to be done. A popular intern's proverb: "The longer you stay, the longer you stay."

If a patient becomes suddenly worse at the end of the day, the intern stays and deals with the problem until the patient is stable, transferred to the intensive care unit, or winds up in the "ECU," the "eternal care unit." In terms of chances for going home, stabilization is worst and requires the most time, while death is best, requiring an hour of attending to various loose ends. To the exhausted and beaten young doc, death is often a favored outcome, not only allowing an earlier escape from the hospital, but meaning there will be one less patient to care for on returning the next day. Another favorite saying of interns: "The best admission is no admission, the next best a dead admission."

Rendered stuporous by lack of sleep, the intern finally staggers home when the day and night and day of on-call ends, and is lucky to get undressed before collapsing unconscious in bed. Some, unable to muster the energy to put the key in the ignition, sleep slumped over the steering wheels of their cars while they sit in the hospital parking lot. The next morning, grizzled and rank after two days without a shave or a shower, they shuffle back in to start the routine all over again.

In most American hospitals, interns "take call" every third day. For example, if the intern is on call Monday, he works through until Tuesday night, crumples at home (or in his car), and returns to work on Wednesday morning. This third day is the only quasi-normal one of the sequence, beginning at 7:00 or 8:00 A.M. and finishing at anywhere from 6:00 to 10:00 P.M. when the day's scut is completed. On Thursday the intern is again on call and works through until Friday evening. Saturday is off and Sunday is another call day, as is the following Wednesday, Saturday, and so on. The average work week of 80 to 120 hours depends on whether there are two or three days of being on call. Some facilities have reduced the call schedule from every third night to every fourth night in an effort to relieve this burden. I suppose it's an improvement, but as far as I'm concerned, slavery is still slavery.

This schedule lasts for a year. When the year is up, the intern becomes a resident. He still "takes" as much on-call, but now supervises scut instead of being the "scutdog."

When asked why this system of medical training exists, hard-nosed American Medical Association types preen and strut like peacocks, gravely announcing, "It gives the boys balls! Teaches them to function under stress!" as though "the boys" were about to assault a beachhead on Guadalcanal.

In fact, the explanation as to why the system exists is very straightforward, and has nothing to do with the reproductive organs of doctors in training. As with much else in the cold, cruel world, it has little bearing on the needs of people. The reason is money, plain and simple.

As though I were trapped in a hideous, never ending cycle of déjà vu, I found myself again on call on the Cloud Pavilion a mere few nights after the Uncle Melvin Show. In fact, the on-call cycle repeated itself with such dizzying rapidity that it seemed I was in the Cloud Pavilion just about permanently. Of course, this wasn't true, and I reminded myself that the time I spent there was no more than 80 to 120 hours a week.

I was in the middle of interviewing another patient when

I got a page from Cloud 8. Because Cloud 8 was not one of the floors I normally worked on, the page probably meant one of the patients I was covering had spiked a temp or crashed or boxed.

"Covering" patients meant being responsible for their medical care at night while their regular interns were at home in a coma. Interns hoped that the patients they covered while on call spent the time sleeping. Many, however, being ungrateful and selfish, insisted on having fevers ("spiking a temp"), or developing some other problem requiring the attention of the covering doc. Those who became very sick "crashed" (becoming "train wrecks"), those who obviated the need for further, time-consuming care died, "boxed," "tubed," and so on.

We had at least a dozen euphemisms for death. Sometimes, when a patient's regular intern returned to the hospital in the morning and inquired of his progress, the covering intern answered by humming taps: "Dum da DUM . . . , dum da DUMMM, dum da DUMM, dum da DUMM. . . ."

On this night some older person whose family had instructed the responsible doctors to treat with fluids and antibiotics *only* (no "heroics") passed away. Rather than being assaulted with the procedure known in the lingo as being "coded," or "teamed," the gentleman simply drifted off. "Coding," or "teaming," was the procedure of administering chest compressions, artificial respiration, and medications designed to reestablish normal activity of the heart. In medical jargon it was called advanced cardiac life support, or ACLS.

This particular patient was found dead and left that way. Bang. As we would say on the Cloud Pavilion, which had only eight floors, the patient "headed for Cloud Nine."

I was paged by a ferociously shy Filipino nurse. She told me she suspected the patient had, uh, passed away, and requested that I come up and declare him. I pursued the conversation in the drunken, uninhibited fashion that came naturally after being awake for twenty hours.

18

"So, you suspect that the patient may be dead, do you?"

"Yes."

"Well, does the patient have any spontaneous respirations that you can detect?"

"No."

"And does the patient have a detectable pulse?"

"No."

"And were you able to get any kind of a blood pressure?"

"No."

"Well, it certainly sounds like the patient is pretty much dead. What do you think?"

"Well, yes, Doctor, but could you please come up and pronounce him dead?"

It was late at night and I was deriving some perverse satisfaction at this torment. The nurse also worked on a floor other than my own. Had she been from my ward she would either have had some fun playing the game or just hung up.

I went up to Cloud 8 to investigate and found that she was right. The patient was dead. I stood next to the bed with the shy and diminutive nurse and said, "Well, I've got to admit it. You were correct. This patient has hallmarks highly suggestive of death. In fact, he is undeniably dead. I declare it, officially." I assumed an air of mock solemnity and addressed the body. "Sir, you are dead. Good luck." I turned around and walked toward the door."

The nurse chimed in before I made good my escape. "Uh, Dr. Intern," she called, her voice nearly inaudible, "please make sure you fill out the death certificate."

Assaulting the elderly and helpless is but one experience of internship that approximates insanity. Anguished, tangled confrontations with a gargantuan array of hospital paperwork occupy an additional 400 percent of the intern's time. As far as the hospital bureaucracy is concerned, the correct completion of paperwork supersedes the survival of the patients themselves. Bungled patients merely die. Bungled paperwork is completed and recompleted until it is letter-perfect.

The patients' charts were crammed with forms. There was the dreaded "M-11-Q, Request for Home Health Services" form, one of the many special treats provided the interns by the department of social services. This form required five pages of fabrication regarding the patient's "home environment," needs for "activities of daily living," and identifying birthmarks of immediate and distant family members. Its completion was necessary if a patient, exhausted and dazed by a prolonged hospital stay, was to receive housekeeping help at home after discharge.

There was the "Medical Summary," requesting in four lines a description of the patient's four-month hospitalization, including "all diagnostic and surgical procedures." This form was often neglected in the frenetic rush to discharge a patient from the hospital; the perplexed intern frequently found himself completing it three or four months later when told to "complete all outstanding charts immediately" if he wished to see his next paycheck. The end of each pay period found the medical records office jammed with befogged interns, each engrossed in wholly imaginary recaps of long-forgotten patients.

There was the form documenting that the patient was offered a Pap smear and detailing the reasons why it may not have been performed. There was the need to cosign all the notes written by medical students. There were the "Request for Consultation" forms, on which consultants in various specialties illegibly detailed their opinions about patients who were headed down the tubes. Each week there was "med renewal day," when the intern arrived an hour early to rewrite the orders for all of his patients.

But, most feared of all, there was the death certificate, an "instrument" (bureaucrat's lingo for a form) used not, as statisticians and administrators might claim, to record the details of an individual's death, but to inflict pain upon interns. It was a form whose correct completion might be taught in a graduate-level university course.

* * *

I froze at the door, the bluster knocked clean out of me.

"Uh, I'm just Dr. Covering Intern. Can't the patient's full-time doc, Dr. Original Intern, complete the death certificate in the morning? After all, he knows the patient better than I do." My eyes pleaded mercy.

The nurse showed no quarter.

"I'm sorry, Doctor, but the hospital requires that the death certificate be completed immediately after the patient expires."

I'd known this all along, but hoped I could deceive my way out of some paperwork. Clearly this tactic wouldn't work. I would have to lie outright. "Okay," I said, "I'll be back shortly." I walked out of the room and headed back to my own floor. Hopefully, the nurse would forget to page me when I failed to return.

She paged me ten minutes later. Disguised in the meek tones of her voice lay the fact that I would have to do battle with the form.

I returned to Cloud 8 and sat at the nurses' station, the dead patient's chart and a blank death certificate on the desk in front of me. I rummaged through my lab coat pockets searching for a pen filled with black ink, in the process accidentally sticking my finger on a used needle whose protective cover had jarred loose sometime over the last ten or twenty hours. Death certificates must be filled out with black ink. I don't know why, but that's the rule. Perhaps any other color is considered inappropriate or distasteful when the subject of record is death.

Naturally, I found no pen in my pockets, despite the cost in blood of the search. I rummaged around the desktop at the nurses' station and asked the desk clerk. Neither produced what I needed. I searched my pockets again, being careful of the now securely recapped used needle. Vaguely, I tried to recall on whom I'd used the needle. I'd stuck at least fifty people since I'd last cleaned out my lab coat pockets. I hoped it didn't come from one of the AIDS patients.

There was not a black pen to be found anywhere on

Cloud 8. I went back down to Cloud 3 and couldn't find one there either. I searched my pockets one last time and, magically, found the black pen that I had thought I was carrying all along. The quest for black ink had consumed twenty minutes, a sum that compared well with the time cost of the first death certificate I'd completed as an intern.

This first encounter had occurred only days after starting internship, on my first or second night on call. A patient had died and, not knowing the black ink rule, I'd faithfully completed the virginal form in blue. A few hours later, at 5:00 A.M., I was paged out of a fitful, sweat-stained, half-hour nap and instructed by a clerk from the death certificate office to recomplete the form in the required, appropriate, tasteful color. Death clerks, entombed in a mysterious office deep in the second or third basement of the hospital, read and filed death certificates, day and night, seven days a week. Their grim task, worthy of a tale by Edgar Allen Poe, was never completed.

Because both the dead patient and, more important, his chart had disappeared hours beforehand, I was obliged to retrieve the certificate I'd already completed from the Death Office and recopy it. Ten minutes of dizzy, near hallucinatory wanderings through basement hallways were required to find the office. There, awash in black pens and crisp, blank death certificates provided by a grimly efficient clerk, I recompleted the form. The clerk surveyed the form and my unsteady, rumpled figure. Finally satisfied, she released me back into the night. The time cost of the whole episode had been over an hour and a half.

I opened the Cloud 8 dead man's chart and referred to the questions on the form. Printing in careful, jet-black letters I recorded the patient's name, and provided the requested, if puzzling, demographic information, certifying, for instance, that the deceased was neither "Hispanic, Not Black," nor a "Pacific Islander." I hoped this would please the Bureau of the Census. Continuing, I boldly declared that I, the M.D. who had pronounced the patient forever dead had, in fact, never actually provided him with medical care.

Next, I encountered the meat of the death certificate, the section intended to detail the cause of death. In bold uppercase letters the first line read, "IMMEDIATE CAUSE OF DEATH."

Since everybody dies of the same thing, i.e., their heart refuses to continue pumping and their lungs likewise pack in the task of breathing, I wrote, with a brashness intended to match that of the question, "CARDIOPULMONARY ARREST."

The following line, entitled "Secondary to, or as a Consequence of," is the trickiest. The uninitiated will not know that there are very specific so-called allowable causes of death, permitted for use on the death certificate.

I assume that the person who originated the concept of "allowable causes of death" was well intentioned, believing specificity in this regard would further the accuracy of statistical studies based on these documents. I've never seen a book listing such illnesses, but assume that it exists. Allowable causes of death, for example, include "lobar pneumonia" or "bronchopneumonia," while simple "pneumonia" is not acceptable. One especially popular among veteran interns is "coronary artery disease."

That night, sitting up on Cloud 8, I was unaware that our patients were refused permission to die, at least on paper, from the diseases they actually suffered. On prior encounters with death certificates I had through sheer luck chosen allowable causes of death.

A quick glance at the present dead patient's chart showed that he'd had a fever and a smudge on his chest X ray. Having boldly declared "CARDIOPULMONARY ARREST" as the immediate cause of death, I now penned, in gentler tones to match the more subdued typeface, that death was secondary to, or as a consequence of, "pneumonia." I signed and dated the certificate, folded it carefully, placed it in an envelope, and launched it into the pneumatic tube system used to rocket messages and other paraphernalia about the hospital.

The task completed, I returned to the nice elderly gentle-

23

man I'd been interviewing before the page. This man was a new patient who was being admitted for a week or two of low-grade temperatures and a cough. My beeper went off again about fifteen minutes into the interview. "Dr. Intern," it screeched, "please call blah, blah, blah, blah." Ominously, blah, blah, blah, blah was the extension of the Death Office. I excused myself from the patient's bedside and answered the page from a phone at the nurses' station.

The Death Clerk answered, "Hello, Death Office."

"This is Dr. Intern," I said, my tone slightly hardened "I was paged."

The Death Clerk, noting my hardened tone and wisely electing not to offer identification, got immediately down to business. "Dr. Intern, you didn't fill out Mr. Deadman's death certificate properly."

My tone hardened further. "What seems to be the problem?"

" 'Pneumonia' is not an allowable cause of death."

"Whaddaya mean 'allowable cause of death'?" I was now slightly puzzled.

" 'Pneumonia' is not listed as an allowable cause of death, Doctor." Extra sarcasm on the word "Doctor."

My tone again hardened. "Well I'm afraid that the patient didn't have the good grace to die of an 'allowable cause of death,' whatever that is. He chose to die of pneumonia, regardless of its degree of acceptability. Unless you wish me to lie and change the form to a listed 'allowable cause of death,' there's very little I can do. Do you want me to lie?"

The Death Clerk's tone was now also hardened. "Whether or not you lie is your business, Dr. Intern [sarcasm again]; the issue, however, is that the death certificate is not acceptable in its present form."

"Well, that appears to be your problem then, doesn't it?"

I hung up and returned to my patient's bedside. He and his wife hadn't budged and still wore the please-be-telling-us-the-truth-that-he-doesn't-have-cancer look. I finished with the history and physical and told the patient and his wife not to worry, that this was only a case of bronchitis, a hair of pneumonia at worst. The patient, I said, would be out of the hospital in three days. I'd almost finished my little speech when the Death Office paged again.

"Dr. Intern," it shrieked, the hardness of voice evident even in the electronic tones of the beeper, "please call blah, blah, blah, blah!" I excused myself once again from Mr. and Mrs. Touch of Pneumonia at Worst and returned to the phone at the nurses' station.

"This is Dr. Intern. I was paged."

"Dr. Intern, you're going to have to come down here to the Death Office and complete this death certificate correctly."

"I thought I made it clear that as far as I was concerned the death certificate was already completed correctly."

"Dr. Intern"—sarcasm peaking—"I told you that pneumonia is not an allowable cause of death."

The edge in my voice began to turn to anger. "Perhaps you'd like to tell me what is an allowable cause of death."

"Lobar pneumonia, Dr. Intern, or bronchopneumonia, Dr. Intern, are allowable causes of death."

"To the best of my knowledge those diagnoses can only be made absolutely definitive at autopsy."

"That may be the case, Dr. Intern."

"I'll tell you what. Have the patient autopsied and when the results are in I'll be glad to run on down and fill out a new death certificate."

I hung up again and returned to my now near hysterical patient and his wife. They appeared certain I had been on the line with their private doc discussing when to start chemotherapy. My beeper went off almost immediately. This time I returned the call from the phone at the patient's bedside, using a tone somewhat more subdued for the benefit of the patient and his wife.

"This is Dr. Intern," I sang. "How may I help you?"

"Dr. Intern, if the death certificate is not completed properly we cannot release Mr. Deadman's body to his family."

There was a sudden surge of bile almost right up to my ears. They were trying, on top of all the other crap I had to deal with in the goddam hospital, to make me feel guilty. I held the phone about a foot from my mouth and, in a voice loud enough to be heard at the opposite end of the hall, yelled, "I told you, dammit, the patient died of pneumonia!" and slammed the receiver. My ears felt hot and red.

I looked up to see my patient and his wife frozen in an attitude of complete and utter terror. I spent the next twenty minutes, a period of time the Death Clerk apparently decided was best left for cooling off, explaining that no, no, no Mr. Touch of Pneumonia at Worst was in no risk of dying. I explained that I'd been talking about another patient, Mr. Deadman, who had multiple complications and a very bad case of pneumonia in no way like that afflicting this patient, and that I sincerely believed he would be back in the bosom of his family in three days at most.

When I stepped outside the room there was a man from administration waiting for me in the hallway. I looked up at him. He had a scrawny beard and wore a badly fitting suit. I knew immediately that he had come to discuss the death certificate. I wondered whether knocking him unconscious would be worth losing my job.

"Dr. Intern?" To my surprise he spoke in a tone clearly meant to be conciliatory.

My belligerence was knocked down a few notches by this fact. I replied in a tired, hostile whisper.

"Yes?"

"Dr. Intern, my name is Mr. Administrator and I've come by because the Death Office asked if I might speak with you about a problem you've been having with them."

This latter "about a problem you've been having with them" established clearly the conciliatory nature of his mission and knocked more steam out of me. That I'd been on my feet for going on twenty-four hours also worked against maintaining any kind of a head of steam. Perhaps this was one of those rare nice-guy administrators who didn't mind treating interns in at least a pseudohuman fashion.

The hostility drained from my voice. "I assume you're speaking about the death certificate."

"Yes. I've taken the liberty of completing a second death certificate in a manner that is acceptable to the Death Office. I've brought along the original that you completed, and if you'll take a moment to compare them you'll see that I've only made a very minor alteration in the 'contributing cause of death.' If it is acceptable to you I'd very much appreciate it if you would sign this second copy."

I examined the administrator's form. Very neatly filled out, it was identical to the one I had completed, but with the addition of the word "lobar" before the word "pneumonia."

The administrator had taken the time to find the best solution to the problem and had done so in the most diplomatic manner possible. A beam of early morning sun appeared on the wall behind him and I started to feel like crying.

I sighed. "That's fine, Mr. Administrator."

I signed the paper and walked away.

Ever since that day I have completed death certificates with "coronary artery disease" as the "contributing cause of death." The Death Office never calls if the cause of death is inaccurate, only if it is unallowable. Virtually every other intern I know does the same, even if the patient died in a plane crash. That's thousands of interns completing death certificates every day. Perhaps this is the reason the United States is now experiencing a statistical wave of coronary artery disease. It is also the reason I have since refused to read medical studies whose findings were based on a review of death certificates.

Mr. Touch of Pneumonia at Worst, by the way, did fine and was discharged from the hospital (via the main entrance rather than Cloud 9) three days later.

2

Never Let Them Make
You Cry

Never, never, never let them make you cry. That was one of my rules on the Cloud Pavilion. And, if they did make you cry, never let 'em see you do it. Don't give them the satisfaction. I only cried once, and it began, naturally, one night when I was on call at the Cloud Pavilion.

I admitted an old guy from home, a patient of one of the private cancer docs (oncologists), for treatment of metastatic (widespread) lung cancer. Saying "from home" was the intern's way of distinguishing that an elderly patient was not from a nursing home and therefore might be somewhere close to being a normal, walking, talking person. Having some functional "squash" or "white matter" locked up in the cranial vault. "From home" was a code phrase implying that more should be done for the patient than for the typical zonked nursing home type who could at best only be returned to a baseline state of low-grade misery.

The old guy who was admitted from home was a nice old guy. He was tall, lanky, bald, and wore round wire-frame glasses. I knew he was doomed as soon as I examined him and felt all the big, fat, cancer-filled lymph nodes sticking out of his neck and armpits, metastases of the lung tumor.

Like a disgruntled army general organizing the overthrow of a banana republic, the tumor had initially established itself quietly and unnoticed in the patient's lung. Slowly it grew, eluding discovery until too late, when, joined by other disgruntled officers, it erupted into action, a gun battle broke out in the military governor's palace, and the patient began to cough up bloody sputum. Squadrons of guerrillas, infiltrated into distant and strategic areas of the country-side, also burst into action at the moment of the coup, blasting ugly lesions into bones, recruiting converts in the lymph nodes, and shooting up holes in random, innocent abdominal organs.

In fact, the moment I met the patient and discovered him to be a nice old guy I suspected he was doomed because of the "conservation of malignancy theory." This theory, held widely by residents and interns, argues that every human being has a given net amount of malignancy in his body. Such malignancy is expressed in two possible ways, through personality or illness. Although in medicine "malignancy" specifically refers to cancer, illness defined by the conservation of malignancy theory includes all debilitating and terminal disease, cancer or otherwise.

The expression of malignancy through personality describes the extent to which a person is a nice guy or an asshole. The more a person is an asshole, the more malignant his personality. This theory is the intern's form of the old maxim, "Nice guys finish last." A nice guy, by virtue of the malignancy lacking in his personality, is much more likely to have an organic malignancy somewhere in his body. Assholes, burglars, and drug peddlers, on the other hand, are so malignant of personality that there is hardly any room for sickness in their bodies.

The conservation of malignancy theory dictates that a nice guy who's lost a bit of weight in the last four or five months has fantastic odds of having a whopping tumor incubating somewhere in his body. Such was the case with Mr. Smith. If he had spent his life as a loan shark, a bagman for the Mafia, or a wife beater, when I ran my hands over his skin looking for swollen lymph nodes I'd have found only smoothness.

Mr. Smith's private doc was Dr. Cancer, one of Manhattan Hospital's hot young cancer jocks. Dr. Cancer was planning on torching Mr. Smith with chemotherapeutic agents designed to battle the malignancy. Although I thought Dr. Cancer was an okay guy, I resented the fact that everybody except the patient himself knew he was going to die regardless of what we did.

"At least we're going to go down fighting," Dr. Cancer had said to me. As I found Mr. Smith to be a gentle, soft-spoken man, I didn't feel good about the idea of using his body for a medical Custer's Last Stand. I also felt awkward when the patient asked what I thought his chances were. I felt he had a right to know the truth but didn't want to interfere with his relationship with his private doc.

I answered with the classic medical hedge: "Well, Mr. Smith, you're a very sick man, the chances of your recovering fully aren't very good and there's no chance of survival without treatment. It's going to be a long and hard road."

This statement was a variation on what I called the Great Medical Hedge. A patient who was very sick, or the family of a patient who was very sick, invariably asked the question, "What will you do for me (or my relative)?" and, "What are my (or my relative's) chances of living?" The Great Medical Hedge was an official-sounding yet vague reply to questions for which we did not have an answer. It cloaked our lack of knowledge in nonspecificity and jargon. It kept us from looking stupid. The Great Medical Hedge went, essentially, "Your chances without treatment are catastrophic, and your chances with treatment are almost as bad, but who knows, you might surprise everyone and live." The statement I had offered Mr. Smith differed from this only in its medicalesque colorings.

Usually, we applied the Great Medical Hedge to those whom we could grab and claw and pull at as they were slowly sucked under. For Mr. Smith, the more honest response would have been, "Well, to tell you the truth, you're sick as a dog and the chances of a cure are about one in a million. The chemicals that are used to treat cancer are more dangerous than what you'd find in the average New

Jersey toxic waste dump. If I were you I'd check out of this dive, withdraw all my money from the bank, and spend it on women and booze, and then give a good long think about whether I was going to chance treatment. Either way, the long-term outcome is going to be the same."

Such honesty would be a problem were the patient to heed it, putting me in the position of having to answer to Dr. Cancer. He'd indignantly demand to know "just exactly what the hell you said to my goddam patient, and just where the hell you thought you got the right to say such a thing." I didn't feel like finding myself in that position. Doc Cancer would get all ruffled up like a cat in heat and go screeching off to the hospital administration and get me in a heap of trouble that I didn't need. The truth is a risky business in medicine.

The thinly disguised dishonesty of the Great Medical Hedge left me feeling anxious and ill at ease. I was relatively smart, eager, and honest, the child of moderately well-off, eggheaded New York City liberals. I'd grown up surrounded by the usual armchair leftist tenets: Poverty was the fault of society, all people were entitled to decent housing, ban the bomb, and blah, blah, blah. Human beings, I was taught, were essentially decent. It was in this setting that I'd come up with the almost unbelievably naïve idea of going to medical school for the archaic purpose of helping people.

Now I was mashed face first into a miasma of ethical contradictions, where the line between helping and hurting, lying and telling the truth, was blurred and distorted beyond recognition. This was a place where the depth of my conviction to be "decent" to people was being tested more bluntly and harshly than ever before. Here, surrounded by shit, vomit, and disinfectant, I tormented Uncle Melvin and lied to Mr. Smith, uncovering shallow areas and uncharted reefs throughout the ocean of my moral psyche.

In fantasies of nobility and strength I'd deal with Doc Cancer's objections to telling Mr. Smith the truth face-to-face, saying, "Well, Dr. Cancer, this one got clean away and you ain't going to get him back no matter what you do to me." The truth is I never faced up to Doc Cancer. He simply arrived one morning, walked into the patient's room, and commenced blasting him with all kinds of garbage.

Back when I was an intern, in the early 1980s, the basic premise in treating cancer was simple. It went, "Kill every last dividing cell in the patient's entire body and hope that the cancer dies before the patient does." The two common modes of therapy, toxic drugs and atom-bomb-type radiation, were based on this premise. Because tumors grow quickly, or, put differently, the cells in tumors divide frequently, interfering with cell division seemed a logical way to kill cancers.

Unfortunately, other, normal cells in the body are also in a constant state of division and renewal. The bone marrow, for example, is normally packed with the precursors of red and white blood cells, busily dividing and maturing before their release into the bloodstream. Cancer drugs blast the bone marrow and render the patient anemic and almost devoid of white blood cells.

White cells, now popularized by all the AIDS press, comprise the immune system, the body's defense against infection. Virtually all cancer treatments at the time I was an intern turned cancer patients into artificial AIDS patients. In the past, docs only saw the bizarre infections now so common in AIDS when they assaulted patients with cancer drugs (a few of which descended from poison gases used during World War I, notably mustard gas) rendering them temporarily immune cripples.

Another area of the body under constant revision and renewal is the gastrointestinal system. The environment inside the stomach is very acidic, and that inside the intestines quite alkaline; both are conditions hostile to cell survival.

The cells that form the lining of the intestines constantly divide and replace themselves. The spectacular puking that follows the administration of chemotherapy probably results from the combined toxic effect of the drug on the GI system as well as a direct effect on the vomiting center in the brain.

In addition to prior attacks with chemo, Mr. Smith had also been prey to radiotherapy, the exposure of that portion of his body victimized by cancer to exploding atom-bomb quantities of radiation. As with chemotherapy, one of the first biologic effects of large doses of radiation is to kill rapidly dividing cells. Radiotherapy is used to treat patients having solid, well-demarcated tumors such as those formed by lung cancer, in contrast to "liquid" tumors, as in leukemia.

Though logical and well reasoned of intent, the actual process of radiation therapy is reminiscent of the machinations of science fiction horror movies. The patient, with the location of the tumor outlined on his skin in bright red crayon, is led into a little room with lead-lined walls, a big, heavy lead door, and a six-inch-wide, twelve-inch-thick lead impregnated window. Hanging from a gigantic spiderlike metal rack suspended from the ceiling is a porcelain-encased doomsday cobalt ray contraption, spirited from the laboratory of a mad scientist. The contraption looks like a deranged torpedo and can be swiveled in all directions on the spider rack to poise the business end directly over the tumor.

The patient is strapped to a stretcher and the cobalt ray tube is positioned two inches over the area marked off in red. Everybody but the patient leaves the room, and the big, heavy lead door swings shut. The machine then begins to hum, indicating the emission of radiation. Outside, the radiotherapists peer in through the lead-impregnated window and gleefully rub their hands. A treatment lasts no more than a few minutes. In that time the patient's nuts, lungs, brain, or whatever organ is victimized by cancer gets fried with more atom-bomb-type radiation than would naturally occur in a million nuclear-weapon-free years.

For perspective, a person whose lung gets irradiated for a tumor might receive several thousand "rads" in "divided doses" over a few weeks; a patient getting a CAT scan ("CAT," incidentally, stands for "computerized axial tomography") gets somewhere on the order of under 10 rads; a chest X ray is worth around a rad, and a brisk walk on a blazing sunny day is measured in thousandths of a rad (millirads).

In my mind's eye the tumor cells quiver and scream and pull their hair out until the radiation ends. There follows a days-long bacchanalian frenzy of murder, rape, and mayhem, and then a strange period of quiet when the cells one by one develop blank stares, cough up blood, have a seizure, and die. The radiation treatments do not kill the patient because the rays are focused on a very small area and are spaced over time.

I think of radiation merely as a kind of pure energy, and envision that it damages tissues and cells by barging in and busting up important and delicate chemical compounds like a bull in a china shop. Radiation medical people (and the Joint Chiefs of Staff) speak of "rads" and "rems," which I vaguely understand as describing the amount of energy absorbed by flesh when it is irradiated. Somewhere also in the dim recesses of my memory is the knowledge that the exposure of one entire person to under 1,000 rads is easily lethal. On the other hand, a small portion of a person can be cooked with many thousands of rads without causing the individual's death, although the involved organ will probably be killed along with the tumor.

While we're discussing the subject of radiotherapy, I might as well put in a plug for atom bombs, also a well-known source of radiation. If an atom bomb happens to go off near a population center, those who survive the immediate heat and blast effects must face the harsh reality of exposure to total body radiation doses on the level of tens of thousands of rads, depending on how close they were to the explosion, in addition to the fact that their local hospital has been rendered a blackened hole in the ground. Most of these people die before their white cells have a chance to disappear. If the dose is big enough, they get the "cerebral syndrome" described in Harrison's *Principles of Internal Medicine* as "produced by acute uniform exposure of the whole brain to several thousand rads and usually fatal. It is characterized by nausea, vomiting, listlessness, and drowsiness followed by tremors, convulsions, ataxia, and death."

If the dose of total body radiation is not large enough to induce the cerebral syndrome, ". . . the gastrointestinal syndrome occurs when the dose of radiation is lower, in the range of 600 to 2,000 rads, and is usually maximal 3 to 5 days after exposure. At the higher doses it is characterized by intractable nausea, vomiting, and diarrhea leading to severe dehydration and vascular collapse."

Untreated, it results in death. For those who don't get a dose big enough to cause these, perhaps being in a Maine wilderness area when the Russkies drop one of their big twenty-megaton babies on New York City, *then* there is the syndrome of white cell death and overwhelming infection.

Like a 1950s movie monster under a hail of police bullets, Mr. Smith's lung tumor had moaned and staggered back under earlier onslaughts of chemo and radiotherapy, wounded but not dead. After sulking and licking its wounds for a few months, it had lunged forward again, its eyes bloodshot with hatred and vengeance for the previous attack. Doc Cancer had readmitted him for a last stand, to "go down fighting."

The only saving grace of the whole deal for my peace of mind was that the drugs were so toxic that Dr. Cancer had to administer them himself. At least I didn't have to do that aspect of the dirty work.

The antineoplastics did nothing more, of course, than hasten the patient's death. Like a boxer being punched senseless, over and over, by a vastly superior opponent, he lay in bed getting blasted by sequential doses, or "runs," of chemotherapy. His "white cell count," the number of white blood cells per cubic millimeter of blood (normally 5,000-8,000), dropped so far as to be almost undetectable; the last of the hair on his already near bald pate gasped its last breath and flung itself onto his pillow; and his body, unable to tolerate food by mouth without overwhelming nausea, gradually wasted into angled gauntness.

The crowning event, the final resolution for Mr. Smith, would be an infection. His body, debilitated and almost devoid of immune defense, was a prime target for a bewildering array of bacterial, viral, and fungal infestation. I reasoned that his junky, tumor-clogged lung provided the most likely site for an infection and checked him on a daily basis for fever, cough, and any new sounds in his chest that might suggest pneumonia.

I was not disappointed. The patient developed a fever almost before Dr. Cancer had finished injecting him with the first round of toxic waste. I immediately wrote an order for him to be given an industrial-strength dose of penicillin and Doc Cancer immediately had the order canceled, saying that the fever was not indicative of infection, but the result of a large number of dead tumor cells being released into Mr. Smith's bloodstream. It was only a side effect of the chemo, he said, and was called tumor fever.

I wasn't buying it. I sent the patient off for a chest X ray and managed to snatch it from the X-ray department before it disappeared forever into the file room. I put it up on one of the light boxes and, lo and behold, there was a new haziness in his lungs, surely proof that he had pneumonia after all. I returned to his chart and rewrote the order for penicillin. When Doc Cancer arrived in the morning, he canceled the order, explaining that the haziness on the chest X ray was not pneumonia, but an entity called pulmonary fibrosis, a stiffening of the lungs, that was also a side effect of the chemotherapy. Furthermore, he explained, the patient already had loads of dead lung in his chest from his radiotherapy treatments; this too would contribute to the haziness. He admonished me not to write orders for his patient without checking with him first and, smiling, left the ward.

I walked into Mr. Smith's room, exasperated. He had a fever again, and was sweaty and coughing and sick as a dog and I couldn't even give him a few palty doses of penicillin. To compound matters, none of his blood cultures had come back positive. Blood cultures were tests I'd done to prove without doubt that he really did have an infection. Whenever he had a fever, I'd stick him with a needle, remove a dollop of blood, and squirt it into a bottle of culture broth. If he had bacteria in his blood, something that was likely if he had pneumonia, they would eat the culture broth, grow strong and robust, and multiply until they could be seen with the naked eye.

I'd become very fond of Mr. Smith and to demonstrate my affection stuck him for a blood culture every time he had a fever in the hopes I'd catch a bug swimming in his bloodstream. So far, all of the cultures, which were cooked for a week in the bacteriology lab, showed "no growth." This was further evidence, as Doc Cancer smugly pointed out, that the patient didn't have an infection after all.

I dragged my resident into the fracas, and he agreed that trying antibiotics couldn't hurt. Together we begged Doc Cancer to let us give the patient a few homeopathic doses of penicillin. Unfortunately, the controversy had developed an ego of its own, and the lines were now firmly drawn. Medical students gathered round, enraptured, as Doc Cancer and his metastatic associates continued to calmly regard the patient's fever and chest X-ray changes as red herrings, while my resident, myself, and a few sympathetic onlookers entrenched ourselves in the theory of infection and pneumonia. As Doc Cancer was the patient's private doc, the big cheese, what he said was the final word, and Mr. Smith continued without treatment.

As the patient continued to deteriorate, the logic of trying

37

antibiotics became glaringly obvious. My resident and I, too fatigued to continue arguing, merely backed off and, after a few face-saving days, Doc Cancer strode briskly onto the ward, announcing, "I think it would now be prudent to administer antibiotics to Mr. Smith," and strode briskly back off again.

Mumbling, "Gee, how come I didn't think of that?" I removed Mr. Smith's chart from the rack and wrote an order for two million units of penicillin IV every six hours, a course approximating half the entire production of the drug during World War II.

Instead of getting better, Mr. Smith merely stopped looking worse, like the boxer being massaged and administered sips of water between rounds of his most brutal fight. His fevers and sweats stopped promptly, his coughing diminished, and his chest X rays froze into an unchanging mess of streaks and shadows.

The patient emerged from this state of medical limbo one week after I started him on antibiotics. Doc Cancer strode back onto the ward and declared, "Mr. Smith has now had an adequate trial of antibiotics. Please discontinue the penicillin order. I will be resuming chemotherapy in the morning." I raised my right hand and rang an imaginary bell suspended in the air. Round twelve would now commence.

As promised, Doc Cancer came along in the morning and administered another blast of chemo to Mr. Smith. He became febrile, diaphoretic (sweaty), and began coughing up a storm in less than forty-eight hours. It was as though no time had passed at all, like the program had been interrupted by a commercial, we'd all gone off for a snack in the kitchen, and, when we had comfortably settled back on the couch, it returned right where it stopped. I resumed stabbing the patient for blood cultures and irradiating him with daily chest X rays. Mysteriously, the blood cultures continued to show no signs of bacteria, though the smudges and streaks on his X rays recommenced their growth. I imagined that by holding the films in a neat stack in front of a light and flipping through them quickly one might see a time-lapse X-ray movie of the development of a pneumonia.

I walked into Mr. Smith's room one morning about four days after I'd written the order to stop the penicillin. He was pale as a ghost, covered with sweat, and running a temp of 104. I was frustrated and confused and angry and tired. His case had become a mess of signs and clues that led boldly toward a conclusion and then faded into nothingness, like a dirt road disappearing into a desert. We could say nothing conclusive about the response of his illness to treatment, about the meaning of his fevers and continued deterioration, about the value of the chemo or the antibiotics. He'd come into the hospital with cancer to be treated and that was exactly what we did, and we'd wound up with a bewildering mess, this poor old bastard who was swirling and rushing down the tubes with catastrophic, terrifying, vicious, relentless, dizzying speed. There wasn't even anyone to blame, not the patient, not myself, not Doc Cancer. There was just this horrifying mess of a man, my patient, bespectacled Mr. Smith.

I sat down on the edge of his bed and asked him how he was doing. He was really sick and had started to lose his marbles because of all of his illness, and all of a sudden he started to talk about how he wanted to have a bowl of ice cream.

I said, "Now where am I supposed to get you a bowl of ice cream?" I figured he'd flipped completely but that I'd play along with him. He was right on the edge of death and had developed incredibly big, shining, lustrous eyes that people sometimes seem to get right before they die.

He said, "You know, there's that guy that sells ice cream down by the entrance to the hospital. You know, right inside the main entrance."

I thought about this for a few seconds and imagined a guy with white pants and a white shirt and a black bow tie with an ice cream cart right near the entrance to the hospital.

I said, "I'm really sorry, Mr. Smith, but there really isn't any such person," but he kept saying, "Yeah, Doc, there's a guy who sells ice cream down there, whyn'cha go and get me a bowl of vanilla ice cream, whaddaya say, Doc?" and I kept insisting that this wasn't true. There we were, this dying guy with great big, shining eyeballs and this poor slob intern sitting on the hospital bed having a discussion about ice cream.

Finally I got up and left the room to go attend to something else. About a half hour later I got a page from the bacteriology laboratory, the people who cook the blood cultures. I called the lab and one of the techs said, "Oh, yeah, Dr. Intern, your patient, lemme see, uh . . . , Mr. Smith. He's got four out of four bottles positive for gram-positive cocci in pairs."

This was definitive medical terminology for, "Mr. Smith has a whopping infection, probably pneumonia." I hung up the phone and called the nurses' station and asked for Mr. Smith's nurse. When she got on the phone I said, "Listen, I know you're busy but I'd really appreciate it if you'd drop everything you're doing and mix up two million units of penicillin and go squirt it into Mr. Smith." She was a nurse whom I got along with and she said, "Okay," and hung up the phone.

Then I ran up the stairs to Mr. Smith's room, pulled open the curtain around his bed, and found him lying there no more than fifteen minutes dead. I just stopped and stood and looked at him and all of a sudden I realized that I'd been right, there was no guy in white pants and a white shirt and a black bow tie selling ice cream at the entrance to the hospital, but there was a coffee shop right there near the entrance with a take-out counter and there was a guy behind the take-out counter who'd be glad to sell you a container of ice cream, and that's what Mr. Smith had been trying to tell me about. In fact, that was exactly what he'd described but for some reason it just didn't get through to

40

me. When the nurse came into the room with the two million units of penicillin, she found him dead and me sitting on the edge of his bed sobbing like a baby, and that was the only time I ever cried when I was an intern.

In retrospect, I realize that I should add for the sake of fairness that not all cancer patients wound up like Mr. Smith. I don't want to, but I know I should. To depict his case as the only way a cancer patient was managed would be a lie. Every once in a while you'd run across a nice-guy oncologist who did not believe in senseless patient torture. The kind of doc who'd shrug his shoulders and talk about "quality time" when the prognosis was undeniably grim. This sugar-coated speech was just a fancy version of what I wanted to say to Mr. Smith. It went, "Forget about treatment because it will just hasten your death, and live fully while you can. There is still quality time left." In many ways I believe this to be better than the go-down-fighting approach, but I also have mixed feelings about the whole thing. Other than the mess-up with his pneumonia, it's not even possible to label Mr. Smith's case as a cut-and-dried example of bad medical care. The fact is that death is a rough pill to swallow, and one cannot judge as right or wrong the decision never to accept it. The worst part was not how he was managed, but how little say he had in his own management. I would have felt much better about the case if the patient had made his own decisions, and based them on a blunt presentation of the facts. But that's not what happened.

That's not what happened with many of the patients on the Cloud Pavilion. It was jammed with Mr. Smiths, people who were sick beyond all promise of recovery but were treated regardless, with a kind of medical machismo, denied the refusal to "go down fighting" despite the cost to the patient or even his clear and informed consent. It was chock-full of Uncle Melvins, hopelessly demented elderly nursing

41

home patients who, lying in bed like sedated laboratory dogs, underwent a dizzying shuttle between nursing home and hospital, hospital and nursing home, until they fell victim to an illness that doctors could not torment them through alive.

As an intern it was my duty to simply shut up and manage the medical details of these patients, and that's exactly what I did. Highfalutin ethical and philosophic discourses were not a part of my job. Nonetheless, by the time Mr. Smith died, a few months into my career as a doctor, I'd developed a sneaking suspicion that hospitals weren't necessarily good places for sick people, that doctors didn't necessarily do good, that something was fundamentally wrong with the whole system. It was a suspicion that would grow stronger as the internship year progressed.

3

The Sundowner and
the Rich Man

Somebody should have told me, way back when I made the decision to become a doctor, somebody should have sat me down and said, "Kid, think twice. It ain't what it seems to be from the outside, this medical business. It has nothing to do with the hype, or the status, or the media image, or Ben Casey, or Marcus Welby, or any of that crap. The fact is that it can get very ugly and very uncomfortable, so give it a good long think before you get involved."

The race to become a doctor begins in high school, where students compete to get into the big-name colleges. Not getting into an Ivy League school is considered a major screwup because the big name is naturally going to be a plus on medical school applications. That was how seventeen-year-old kids were thinking when I went to high school, at the bitter end of the late 1960s early 1970s, the we-can-change-the-world era, when kids still wore bell-bottoms. High school and college kids today are much more openly career-minded and interested in money, and I hear the exact same competitive sentiments.

43

The real cutthroat competition for getting into medical school begins in college. Med schools require a certain degree of science education, so much chemistry, math, physics, and the like, the more of everything the merrier. Most colleges offer only one of each of the premed courses per semester. For this reason, being premed (a derogatory title) means being stuffed into classes with all the other premeds. Each engages in a life-and-death struggle for grades that can result in seriously deranged behavior.

Many professors "teach" courses not to impart knowledge but to weed out the weaker premeds in a distorted intellectual process of Darwinian natural selection. A chemistry prof at my college put triple-negative wording on exam questions. Occasionally he'd throw in a question on a subject he had mentioned in class that had nothing to do with chemistry. If someone complained he'd explain that everything said in class was intended as teaching. A true jerk.

College continues in a similar fashion. Students grow bags under their eyes from spending Saturday nights studying in the library, sabotage one another's chemistry lab experiments, lace class notes with misinformation to be fed to colleagues, and spend exorbitant amounts of money on standardized test review courses, all the essential ingredients of the well-rounded liberal arts education. Some students gild medical school applications by cultivating unique outside interests, like the ability to play the ukelele or dance the rhumba. Others become immersed in some infinitesimally small detail of research being conducted at the university's biology department. Like schoolboys in love, they daydream of seeing their names recorded in the microscopically fine print of esoteric scientific publications like *The American Journal of Cell Wall Synthesis,* or *Amino Acid.* Volunteer work at a local hospital provides standard summer fare. Here, surrounded by blood, death, and haggard, hollow-eyed doctors, the student comments on the "fascinating work" and "intellectual stimulation" so inherent

44

in medicine.

Finally, the student is ready to apply to medical school. At the cost of a mere twenty or thirty bucks a shot, applications are sent to all the medical schools in the Northern Hemisphere, including a few "safety schools" in Mexico or the Caribbean. There follows an Alka-Seltzer and Maalox drenched period of waiting for interview invitations. Those unlucky enough to make it through this step next rush out to purchase an interview suit, drain their parents' credit cards purchasing plane tickets, and have their hair cut.

For those with catastrophically bad luck, the black letter arrives sometime in the fall semester of the senior year. In the first ever act of generosity to fellow premeds, the student who is admitted to one or more institutions diligently withdraws all applications from lesser preferred schools.

I began my premed career with similar pathology, arriving at my dormitory room after late nights in the library to find PLEASE KNOCK signs on the door, indicating that my roommate was inside humping his girlfriend. I'd sneak the key in the lock and fling open the door, screaming "I'm coming in!" while his girlfriend shrieked. That was about the most fun I had in my early premed career.

I began to burn out early in the junior year, initiating an academic slide that has yet to abate. Saturday nights in the library were transformed into embarrassing, intoxicated, and mostly futile attempts to avoid total celibacy. I spent my summers hitchhiking around the country, and left the local hospital to take care of itself.

Despite this scarred and chaotic career, I discovered in myself the ability to be "clutch" on exams. My med school applications fused relatively high grades with a dash of the vagabond, a combination that proved intriguing to admission boards. I interviewed at Manhattan University Medical College with a short, fat doc who chain-smoked, filling the tiny interview room with a gray haze. He looked at my application and, noting that I'd thumbed to Alaska, got all excited. He'd spent a few years there and loved it. We spent the entire interview talking about traveling, as though we were bullshitting in a bar. At the end he looked at his watch, told me we were out of time, and said, "Well, I assume you want to be a doctor for all the right reasons."

I said, "I hope so," not knowing at all what he meant, and got into the school a few weeks later.

I decided on MUMC because it was a few blocks from Central Park, a great place for jogging. This was, in fact, the factor that made me happiest there and, ever since, I've used the quality of local jogging facilities as the number one criterion in choosing a job or place to live.

One day, while I was on short call on Cloud, I admitted an elderly man named Horace Kram. At Manhattan Hospital being on "short call" meant admitting a maximum of three patients until three in the afternoon. Short call was designed to give the people on long call, the poor slobs scheduled to be up all night, a bit of a break during the day. By not starting to take admissions until the afternoon, they'd have a chance to look after the patients they already had in the hospital. For those of us not on long call, chomping at the bit to get the hell out of the hospital, it meant the three possible admissions would roll in from the ER at two-thirty in the afternoon so we'd get stuck until nine or ten working them up. Complain, complain, complain.

Mr. Kram, the ancient gentleman I admitted, was sent up to a bed on Cloud 5, a floor set aside for patients who were not acutely ill, those more in need of a "tune-up" than a cure. Patients on Cloud 5, being theoretically not so sick, were supposed to require minimal intern care. The patients' private docs were to write most of the orders, decide on discharge, and so on.

Usually, of course, such patients were grotesquely ill, and required not only a great deal of care from the intern and resident, but also the completion of eight zillion forms necessary for transfer to a regular full-care floor.

My resident and I walked into one of the four-bedded rooms. As was often the case with the very old and very sick, Mr. Kram lay in bed curled up like a pretzel, totally unresponsive. As with a dried-up crab on the beach, the shaking of one of his limbs, a motion made to further assess his level of consciousness, caused his whole body to move as a single unit, as though his joints had long since rusted shut. Noxious stimuli—poking, pinching, and shaking—did not elicit even a groan from the patient, whose fetally posed form appeared to be another in a long succession of the living dead.

My resident instructed me to place an intravenous line and write admitting orders. Later, we would reconnoiter and decide on a further plan of action.

I stuck an IV into Mr. Kram's tissuelike veins and traipsed off to write his orders. Admitting orders follow a general framework, which includes the patient's diagnosis, meds, routine labs, general condition, allowable level of activities, diet, etc. Mr. Kram's would contain such helpful and useful instructions as "activities: bed rest with bathroom privileges," and "diet: low salt/kosher."

When I finished, I wandered off to attack another patient, some poor soul whose IV had come out, was leaking, hurting, or, for whatever reason, needed replacement. As an intern I spent more time messing about with IVs than monks do meditating. In a single thirty-six-hour on-call shift I'd often place twenty or more IVs.

While prodding the next patient looking for a good vein to punch I suddenly realized that I'd left Mr. Kram's IV wide open. I'd forgotten to close down the little doojiggy that controls the rate of flow on the IV tube, allowing fluid to pour unrestrained into the patient's pretzeloid form. Because one of Mr. Kram's myriad admitting diagnoses was "congestive heart failure," I worried that an impromptu liter of IV fluid would completely overfill his arteries and veins, tax his aging heart, and wind up sloshing around in his lungs, a process called fluid overload.

I zipped down the hall and up the stairs to Mr. Kram's room and stopped dead on arriving at his bedside. The IV bag hung completely empty above the patient, who was sitting up in bed with his legs crossed and his face hidden by a newspaper.

Mr. Kram, apparently, had been a bit dry. "A bit dry" (intern's slang, the more proper medical phrase being "dehydrated") meant the patient was all dried up and shriveled like someone who'd spent a few days without water in the desert.

Very frail old people are easily dried out. When kept from taking water for just a day they prune up completely. Even worse, many such folks take peeing pills (medical term, "diuretics"; popular, "water pills"), which are useful in a wide variety of medical conditions. There are several dozen different types of diuretics, of which two or three fit into a category of drugs I fondly referred to as "drugs that actually work." Listed in the *Physician's Desk Reference,* or *PDR,* the industry standard, are literally thousands and thousands of meds. Among them there are perhaps two dozen, fifty at most, "drugs that actually work."

In the United States there are better than several million people taking diuretics on a daily basis, the vast majority of whom are old folk. If an old person on a diuretic gets to feeling a little bit under the weather and doesn't drink anything for even half a day, the very delicate balance between too much water and too little gets upset. The patient can dry up and gork out in a matter of hours. This is not surprising given that even a healthy person will prune if forced to lose water without drinking. A healthy young adult, for example, who sweats like a dog on a hot day in July and is then deprived of water gets weak and groggy in no time. Pissing pills are akin to forced sweating on a hot day in July except that they force water loss through the kidneys.

In addition to the fact that Mr. Kram was on big-time

48

diuretic doses, it happened to be on a hot day in July that we admitted him. He'd probably been sweating up a storm, too. Poor guy. It was no wonder he'd looked like a pretzel when he came in and perked up like a drooped daisy with an impromptu liter of saline.

One of Mr. Kram's other admitting diagnoses was "OBS" ("organic brain syndrome"), a nondescriptive, nonspecific medical term that was often applied to old people who thought or acted a little funny. I included OBS in the class of "garbage dump" diagnoses, technical-sounding bits of medical jargon that provided little insight into a patient's real problem. The correct term for the syndrome that afflicted Mr. Kram is "dementia," a precisely defined entity that is frequently the cause of bizarre behavior in the elderly (and, often, the not so elderly). Popularly, dementia is referred to as senility, but this also is poorly defined and used. It is simply the vernacular for the same older-person misbehavior ascribed by doctors to OBS.

Simply put, dementia is a syndrome that affects the cognitive, or higher, functions of the brain, such as memory, judgment, abstraction, and speech. Initially, its effects on immediate and recent memory are most obvious. The afflicted individual finds himself misplacing common items, forgetting about food placed in the oven, etc. As the disease progresses, the memory loss becomes more severe. The patient may fail at work, get lost in a familiar neighborhood, or be unable to recognize an acquaintance. Eventually, a dementia may become severe, or "dense." Memory is almost nonexistent (as with Uncle Melvin, who'd ceased struggling and lapsed into a vacant stare as soon as I stopped his torture), and the other cognitive functions fail, including speech, orientation in time and space, judgment, and abstraction. Despite this, the patient remains fully alert. Severely demented patients wind up lying in bed, wide-awake, staring numbly at the ceiling and collecting bedsores.

There are several different kinds of dementia. Examples

include Alzheimer's dementia, senile dementia, multi-infarct (lots of strokes) dementia, and pseudodementia. Also, a number of drugs and medical conditions (being dried up like a prune, for example) can cause or compound a dementia, which disappears if the drug is removed or the medical problem treated. Other conditions mimic dementia. Depression, which is relatively common in the elderly and causes similar cognitive problems, is one such condition. Delirium (most often resulting from head trauma, severe medical illness, or drug or alcohol ingestion) creates clouding of consciousness and an altered perception of physical reality (an "altered sensorium") that can also resemble dementia.

The severity of a dementia is investigated with the "mental status exam," a series of questions that test cognitive skills. Immediate memory, for example, is tested by asking the patient to repeat a spoken phrase, and long-term memory by asking him where he lived as a child. The patient's ability to make simple, logical decisions (what would he do if he found a stamped, sealed envelope lying on a sidewalk?) implies sound judgment, while his capacity to interpret proverbs (e.g., "A rolling stone gathers no moss") explores abstraction. As simple as this test sounds, I was often surprised by its results. The number of people who elected to leave the envelope on the ground, burn it, open and read its contents, or drop it in a garbage can was frightening, and subsequently caused me to grasp my correspondence with an iron fist on the way to the mailbox. Others interpreted proverbs literally ("Rocks have to sit still for moss to grow on them"). This concreteness was another sign of dementia.

Often, demented patients recognize their problem and feel embarrassed by it. Understanding this is important to the investigator, who may put the patient at ease by asking easily answered questions such as queries about the distant past, before slowly and gently probing into confusing inquiries about what happened five minutes ago or last week.

Being a voyeur about the details of people's lives, I loved to ask people questions about themselves. Many of the patients at Manhattan Hospital were elderly Eastern Europeans who had emigrated to the United States in the last century. They grew up in a different world.

They'd say, "Well, I came to this country when I was seven years old from a village named such and such in Poland. That was in 1897. We lived in the Bronx for many years before my parents died. You should've seen the Bronx back then. It was mostly farmland."

Then I'd ask, "Do you know what today's date is?" If they were good and demented the answer was off by at least ten years.

I took care of one lady who was 104 years old and had a very mild dementia. Every morning when I went into her room she'd ask me the same question, "Do you know why I lived to be so old?".

I'd say, "No, why?" and she'd say, "It's because Hitler fed us straw." She'd spent the Second World War in concentration camps and was convinced that eating straw to keep from starving to death was the reason for her longevity.

This exchange inevitably prompted the memory that her entire family had been slaughtered by the Nazis and she would break down in tears even now, over forty years later. Soon, I learned to head off these memories. When she asked, "Do you know why I lived to be so old?" I'd say, "Yes, Mrs. Cohen, it's because Hitler fed you straw, and how are you feeling this morning?" Mrs. Cohen's dementia was typically mild; her memory included the horrors of her youth, but not the fact that she'd asked me the same question only one day before.

Mr. Kram had a serious case of dementia, though it was not yet "dense." He had lost his grip on the present and recent past so thoroughly that he lived almost permanently in the far past. Just about every time he saw me he'd go on about how he knew me years earlier. I was his former card partner, a buddy of his in the army, an associate of his when he was in the garment business, an in-law. He had absolutely no idea that he had seen me just the day before, and when he wasn't convinced we were longtime associates he'd say, "And what's your name, Doc?" He knew nothing of who the president was, what the date was, and whether or not the place he was in was a hotel or a hospital.

Sometimes when I was on call I'd stop by his room to check in on him. I'd stand for a moment, listening to his oblivious, quiet mumbling, and find myself wishing that I was wherever it was that he was, like having a cup of coffee with his cronies at the automat down in the garment district in 1956, rather than on call at Manhattan Hospital.

In my experience with old people, I found little investigation into the cause of "senile" behavior. Somewhere along the way addled old folks simply picked up the label "OBS." To me OBS came to mean, "This person has some sickness in his brain that makes him think and act funny, though no one has seriously set about determining what exactly that sickness is." It was like admitting a patient with a chronic cough and calling it organic lung syndrome. Whereas no one would ever accept the statement, "Well, the patient has a sickness in his lungs that's caused a chronic cough but no one's really bothered to look into it," the term "OBS" didn't seem to be a problem. The sad part about it was that several of the causes of OBS were treatable. A babbling, drooling old person sometimes reverted to near normalcy. Regardless, few of the old folks I admitted carrying a diagnosis of OBS had records of a dementia work-up.

Mr. Kram was one of those few. Fancy X-ray specialists had peered at fancy X rays of his head, blood experts had poked and prodded and tested his blood, brain docs had studied chicken scratch recordings of his brain waves. He'd even had an intern stick a needle into his spine and suck out a little sample of spinal fluid for testing on the off chance that a moment's indiscretion in his youth had led to a syphilitic infection of his nervous system.

Finally, the X-ray docs won out. Pointing and gesticulating at X rays and CAT scans displayed in dark rooms on brilliant light boxes, they indicated the alarming amount of shrinkage that had occurred in Mr. Kram's brain over the years. It was decided that he'd had so many little strokes that there was no longer enough working brain tissue in his head for him to think properly. He had multi-infarct dementia.

In all likelihood, Mr. Kram's dementia, his "senility," had been a contributing factor in his becoming dried up like a salted snail. Possibly he was feeling thirsty at the nursing home but, because of the compounding effect of increasing dryness on his dementia, he may have asked for a deck of cards instead of a glass of water. Perhaps a few hours later, an hour or so before they found his arid, bed-bound form, he'd asked for a bag of nails, also meaning to convey his need for a glass of water. A nurse at the nursing home may have commented, "Poor Mr. Kram, he's just about lost the last of his marbles."

An hour later, his brain now almost completely freeze-dried, he'd been unable to ask for anything and was shunted off to Cloud, advertised on the "Nursing Home Transfer Summary" as "rule-out CVA." There, inadvertently, a fatigued and slightly careless intern, almost a recent high school graduate, filled him back up with fluid, cooling his radiator and solving the problem accidentally and unknowingly.

That the patient was demented did not mean that he was not a charming guy. He put down his newspaper when I came into his room. A pair of black horn-rimmed glasses that hadn't been washed for at least a year sat on a truly gigantic nose. His lips, cheated of flesh for use in the

53

construction of his nose, stretched themselves into an expression of surprised pleasure. His eyes lit up.

"Doc!" he cried. "Jeez, how the hell are you? How the hell long's it been anyway? Christ! It must be twenty-five years. Hell, those were some damn times we used to have, weren't they?"

I could only regard the patient with a dumbfounded grin. He continued to smile at me, his head tipped back to allow him to peer through the filthy glasses, which had slipped down his enormous nose.

"Ah, Christ, Doc!" he exclaimed. "Yeah, you always were a quiet one." He waved a hand at me and resumed his intent study of the paper.

I stood for several seconds staring at Mr. Kram with my mouth open, trying to determine what exactly had happened and then ran off to call my resident. I told him in the most serious voice I could muster to come up and see Mr. Kram as soon as possible. He wanted to know if the patient had died already. I said no, and asked him again to hurry up as soon as possible.

I waited for him in Mr. Kram's room, where I had pulled the curtain around the patient's bed for dramatic effect. When he came in I pulled it open with a flourish, revealing the pretzelman transformed into a living, breathing, newspaper-reading older gentleman. My resident stood gawking as I had and commented on how a little fluid could work wonders.

That was the last time I had any fun with Mr. Kram. His heart, weak, ornery, and cranky, worked as though it were a vast piece of scar tissue with two remaining functioning myofibrils. Myofibrils are the little muscle cells that pull and relax, pull and relax, pull and relax ceaselessly in the lifetime of a heart. Mr. Kram's myofibrils had been dying one by one since the Harding-Coolidge era. The death of so much working muscle had weakened his

54

aging heart to the point that it had gotten saggy and weak and was no longer able to pump scads of blood as it had when it was youthful and robust. Being dilated and tired, no longer a sleek pumping muscle, it had started to fail.

To further explain Mr. Kram's alarming condition it is first necessary to understand some basic human anatomy (structure) and physiology (function). The heart is really just a glorified pump. Blood delivers its load of oxygen to the busily living tissues of the body, collects waste carbon dioxide produced by those same tissues, and passes through millions of yards of veins into the vena cava (one of the "great" blood vessels), and the right side of the heart. The right side of the heart (which is comprised of two "chambers," the right atrium and right ventricle) then contracts, delivering the now tired, blue-tinged, and oxygen-choked blood to the lungs.

Once in the lungs, the blood enters jillions of fantastically tiny blood vessels called capillaries (these are so small that the red corpuscles must pass through single-file) that surround air bags called alveoli. There are so many jillions of blood vessels and air bags that the few ounces of blood pumped by each heartbeat are dispersed over a surface area equal to a tennis court. The blood then absorbs whatever happens to be in the alveoli, usually a combination of cigarette smoke, air pollution, and oxygen, and releases its load of waste carbon dioxide.

Bright red, oxygenated, and raring to go, the blood now shunts to the left side of the heart. Here it passes from the left atrium to the left ventricle, which gives it a great huge heave that plummets it into another of the body's "great" blood vessels, the aorta, and begins a new circuit. Occurring at a rate of sixty times per minute in a lifetime of seventy years, this process is repeated over two *billion* times.

Listened to with a stethoscope, the pumping heart goes "lub-DUP!" For me, the symmetry of the human body and rigid logic of medicine have a beauty that has survived and transcended the sham of medical training.

Mr. Kram's heart had lost this sleek efficiency somewhere around the beginning of Eisenhower's second term. Like any failing pump, the fluid it was meant to move backed up and overflowed into the wrong places. His left ventricle, baggy and dilated rather than streamlined and powerful, was simply unable to keep up with all the blood delivered to it from the lungs. Blood backed up into all the jillions of fantastically small blood vessels around the air bags in his lungs. As the pressure built up, fluid from the blood wept and oozed out into the little air bags, turning them into fantastically small water bags.

Gradually, more and more air bags would fill with fluid and Mr. Kram would get more and more short of breath. He'd shriek, "Help! I'm drowning!" and that was exactly what was happening. When I put my stethoscope to his back I'd hear all the fluid sloshing around and bubbling and gurgling in his lungs every time he took a breath.

Because his right ventricle had also failed, blood backed up into his millions of yards of veins as well as into his lungs. His neck veins, engorged with blood, stood out like they did on Louis Armstrong when he played the trumpet. Blood backed up for miles, right down to his feet. Here, as it had done in the lungs, fluid seeped out of the blood vessels into the surrounding area, causing his ankles to swell up. Grabbing his ankle and squeezing left a soft, squished-out handprint, as though his flesh were actually Silly Putty.

A patient who is short of breath and has sloshing, bubbling lungs, bulging neck veins, and puffy, Silly Putty ankles, is said to have congestive heart failure, or CHF. This really means the backing up and slopping out of the blood into all the wrong places resulting from a failing heart. If the patient is really short of breath and blue in the face, medical terminology focuses on the lungs and the condition is called acute pulmonary edema, which means sudden sogginess of the lungs.

Mr. Kram had one hell of a case of CHF. His heart was

mostly one gigantic piece of scar tissue. There was only a very precise amount of blood he could tolerate. If his blood volume went just an ounce over he became "fluid overloaded," his heart screamed that it couldn't keep up with the pumping, and fluid leaked out all over the place, in his lungs, his neck veins, his feet. He'd get short of breath from acute pulmonary edema and tell the nurse, who'd page me and say, "Mr. Kram says he's short of breath."

I'd come running when one of the nurses told me someone was short of breath because I was afraid they might stop breathing and die. In contrast, I wouldn't come nearly so quickly when told someone had a fever because people don't kick off in a matter of seconds from a fever. When I arrived at Mr. Kram's bedside and put my stethoscope at his back, I'd hear all the fluid in his lungs bubbling and gurgling. I'd go to the medication room, fill up a syringe with Lasix, one of the more popular diuretics, and go squirt it into his intravenous line. Within a half hour Mr. Kram would begin to pee all over his bedclothes, as Lasix is a very powerful pee drug. The object of doing this, other than giving the nurse's aide extra work to do, was to cause the patient to pee out a bunch of water, reduce the volume of his blood (which is made of blood cells, proteins and other molecules, salts, and water), ease all the congestion, and allow the backed-up fluid to seep back out of the air spaces into the blood vessels where it belonged. Shortly, Mr. Kram would stop feeling short of breath.

One of the problems with caring for Mr. Kram was the difficulty of making him pee off the exact right amount of fluid and not pee himself right back into his initial pretzel-form state of dehydration. His heart was not only extremely sensitive to too much fluid but also to too little. If he peed off a half liter too much his heart wouldn't be able to maintain a blood supply to all of his body organs and he'd prune out in a matter of minutes. The only time I saw him in a perfectly balanced state was that first day when I accidentally dumped a liter into him over a period of five minutes. For the rest of the month or so that I had him as a patient he'd either be dripping like a soaking-wet sponge or dry like a saltine cracker. A hair too much fluid and he'd go floating and gurgling off down the hallway and a hair too much Lasix and he'd dry up and gork out in just a few hours.

In addition to being demented, Mr. Kram was also what was known to interns as a "sundowner." The onset of darkness would confuse him to the point that he became little more than a baby. Like an ornery infant he'd stay up all night, shitting, babbling, and screaming for attention. Late at night he could be heard from down the hall yelling, "Help me, help me!!" Going into his room did no good, he'd persist in shrieking, "Help me, help me!" even when I stood at his bed telling him to relax and shut up. His roommates were driven to a near homicidal state by this behavior. Finally, I managed to get him a private room. When the sun went down I quietly shut the door and left him to live out the nightmares that would shortly possess him.

Despite his dementia he learned to use the call buzzer, the button at the bedside that patients use to call for a nurse. In this way he was not abandoned completely at night. He'd buzz and buzz and buzz, hundreds of times a night, driving the nurse insane instead of his former roommates.

Eventually I tired of taking care of Mr. Kram. Though still new at the job, I'd learned a variety of patient-dumping tricks and got rid of him by telling the social worker that he was no longer in need of "acute care" and could be transferred to the "chronic care" section of the hospital. The chronic care section looked after people who were no longer in need of a regular floor bed but weren't stable enough to be shipped back to the nursing home. It was a

58

kind of medical purgatory, with a disinfectant- and shit-scented "rec room" with card tables and board games surrounded by old folks slumped over in their wheelchairs.

I made sure to arrange for Mr. Kram's transfer at one of those rare times that his fluids were just about perfectly balanced. I knew it would be only a matter of a few hours before he was too wet or too dry and they'd have to transfer him back to the acute care section. For this reason I planned for the transfer to occur near the end of a day when I was not on call. I held my breath while they shipped him off the floor. Once he was gone I bolted from the hospital. By the time he would need treatment I'd be home, the batteries safely removed from my beeper to prevent any possibility of my being paged.

Cruel but true. When I arrived in the hospital the next day Mr. Kram was back in the Cloud Pavilion, but no longer my patient. One of the other poor bastard interns, someone who was on call the night before, took him as an admission when he was transferred back. He was no longer my problem. Mr. Kram was still there when I finished my rotation on Cloud and I never saw him again.

Mr. Kram kept me busy while he was my patient in the Cloud Pavilion. He kept me much busier than Mr. Cloud, the man who'd donated the money to build the Cloud Pavilion.

Mr. Cloud was admitted to his namesake Pavilion one day so that his private doctors could busily do absolutely nothing for him. He became my patient during the same brutally hot summer, early in internship, that I admitted Mr. Kram, and wound up in a room just out of earshot of the ancient sundowner's nightly hallucinations. He was an elderly man who headed a proverbially vast industrial empire and who, quite out of the blue, one day began to talk in serious tones about committing suicide. In medical jargon such talk is called suicidal ideation. If the patient had been anybody but a major hospital benefactor, he would have been committed to a psych floor. Having bought and paid for Cloud, Mr. Cloud was simply moved in for "medical reasons." This saved his family any embarrassment that might result because its patriarch had gone crazy.

Mr. Cloud's fortune had originated in Europe and I heard a story that he'd gotten himself, his family, and a good chunk of his money successfully out during the war by paying off the Nazis, as he was Jewish. That he had successfully outwitted the most malevolent, vicious group of humans ever to grace the face of the planet impressed me. On arrival in the United States his business savvy told him to immediately change his name—after all, anti-Semitism was not limited to the Nazis—and to donate a ton of his remaining money to a "charitable cause," any favorite of the American monied class. Historically, his plans were spot on. There was a time when the building of hospitals was a moral obligation, and therefore a business necessity, of the wealthy in America.

Being a patient of high status at Manhattan Hospital, Mr. Cloud was admitted to a private room right next to the nurses' station, a class place to be where a scream for help might actually be heard. In further recognition of his status the president of the hospital had a continual stream of concerned-looking bureaucrats marching in and out of his room with gigantic bouquets of flowers and boxes of candy at all times of the day and night. In addition, a group of three or four absolutely gorgeous young women took shifts hanging around outside his door. I suspected the president of the hospital had a group of his yes-men scour the entire institution looking for the prettiest secretaries, who were then pulled from their normal jobs and paid double time to give Mr. Cloud's scowling visage the eye whenever he was wheeled out of his room for a test. The presence of those women while Mr. Cloud was in the hospital made it difficult for the male interns to get any work done at all.

Mr. Cloud's case was attended by a battalion of department heads and specialists, the best the hospital had to offer. His private doc was the head of general (or "internal") medicine at Manhattan Hospital, one of these guys who'd been in the business for about fifty years and had written seven textbooks. He coordinated the patient's care, and attended to the medical details of his case. The head of neurology did his neuro consult, and the head of psychiatry did his psych consult. He had so many specialists and consultants on his case that I had absolutely nothing to do except order the occasional blood test, chase down an X ray or two, or send him for some esoteric examination.

On Cloud, the very best admission was no admission, the next best a dead admission, and the last, an admission like Mr. Cloud that required almost no work. Every day I'd go to his chart and write, "Patient's complaints and physical exam unchanged, progress as per consult notes."

That Mr. Cloud had such conspicuous, high-octane medical muscle in charge of his case was further evidence of his stature in the hospital. At Manhattan Hospital, as at virtually every other private medical institution in the country, it was the department heads, the truly big-cheese private docs, who had the final say in virtually all aspects of hospital policy. It was their status and power in the "medical community" as a whole, their political clout, that sucked ever increasing sums of research, growth, and development money into the hospital coffers. Each headed an army of other private docs in each of the specialties: internal medicine, surgery, obstetrics and gynecology, and so on. They were both master and servant to the private docs, and each policy decision they made helped perpetuate the system of "fee for service," the age-old basis of private medical practice.

Medical costs break down into several categories: the fees doctors charge for their services, the cost of hospitalization (including room and board, X rays, medical equipment used in a patient's care, medications, etc.), specialized laboratory services (such as pathology), and outpatient medications. Until recently, all of these services were paid for on an as-you-go basis, so many dollars for each X ray, office visit, IV, and so on. The vast majority of docs base their charges on this fee-for-service principle, billing for all office and hospital visits, specialized procedures (like surgery or fancy diagnostic procedures), and consultations. Sources of payment include the insurance companies, the government via Medicare or Medicaid (these sources of payment comprising "third-party reimbursement"), or the patients themselves ("out of pocket" payment). Any suggestion of cutting the cost of medical care through fee setting, prepayment plans, or, God forbid, paying docs a set salary, was anathema to the private doc.

The onset of "diagnosis-related groups," or "DRGs," in the early 1980s set off a hullabaloo in private medicine just short of a revolution. The government, responding to a rate of increase in medical costs far greater than inflation, announced that hospitals would be reimbursed for Medicare patients on a diagnostic basis, instead of fee-for-service. Rather than paying for each of the services and procedures provided by the hospital, each patient was worth a given sum based on the admitting diagnosis. A man admitted with a diagnosis of pneumonia, for example, might be worth a set fee of $1,500 under DRGs, while in the past Medicare was billed for however many services the patient received, every X ray, blood test, and so on. Before DRGs, it was in the hospital's financial interest to let a patient hang around, undergoing test after test and piling up bills. Now, they have an incentive to boot the patient out as quickly as possible, preventing the DRG fee from being eaten up in overhead costs.

The bureaucrats who administer DRGs explain that the reimbursement rates represent "average" costs for a given diagnosis, and insist that they will increase efficiency at a time when health care resources are not limitless. Docs, naturally, have become extremely red in the face about the whole thing, declaring that the hospitals' fear of losing money will force them to engage in the wholesale dumping of patients when the cost of their care exceeds the DRG reimbursement rate. Nonetheless, the DRG concept of hospital reimbursement is spreading, and private insurance companies may soon join the feds in adopting it. There are even ominous rumblings of paying docs through a DRG system as well. The AMA will shriek and howl and throw itself on the floor, tearing its hair out and holding its breath until it turns purple before allowing this to happen, but the writing is on the wall.

Medicare, by the way, is the federal health insurance program for people aged sixty-five and over. It has two parts, one covering hospitalization and one for doctor visits. Although DRGs have not yet been applied to the latter, the government does not provide the private docs with a blank check. They are paid via "modified fee for service"; the doc goes ahead and charges for everything he does, and when the government receives the bill, it reduces the payment for some of the services, and refuses to pay for others. Again, reimbursement rates are supposed to represent the average for a given service in a given area. Unfortunately, many, many docs in this country refuse to accept Medicare assignment and bill the patient for whatever the government doesn't pay. When asked why, they will explain that the reason for doing this is that Medicare doesn't cover overhead, never mind allow for a profit. Regardless, for those who are poor, these additional charges can be catastrophic.

In its essence, the medical establishment functions first and foremost to serve the financial interests of the private doc. The AMA criticizes DRGs for changing the focus of medical care from concern for the patient to concern for the bottom line, but one senses that patient care would not change one iota if all docs chose good medicine over continued profits in the now reduced medical resources pot.

At MH, and at all other private hospitals, the private doc, or "attending" (known in intern's slang as "offending") stood at the top of the pecking order. Patients admitted to the hospital by the attendings were assigned to a housestaff team, consisting of a supervising resident, a doc in training who'd already completed the internship year, and two interns. Each of the interns cared for up to fifteen or more patients, and was directed by the resident, who in turn consulted with the patients' private docs regarding details of care. Each team also had an attending with whom they met on a daily basis for rounds: general guidance and teaching about all of the team's patients. Most hospitals required private docs to spend a certain number of months each year acting as a team attending. In return, the private docs were given admitting privileges, allowing them to admit their own patients to the hospital.

The pecking order in the hospital, therefore, went: department head, private doc, resident, intern. The intern was always at the bottom of the ladder. Occasionally, a medical student ("stud" or "scut-puppy") was added to the team. Despite the fact that students were behind interns in years of training, they were above them on the ladder. "Shit rolls downhill," and interns were always at the bottom. They were below the nurse's aides and volunteers at the hospital, below security officers, head nurses, administrators, and laundry room workers. They were below gonorrhea germs growing in a culture dish. They were truly the lowest form of life in the hospital.

Mr. Cloud's private doc, the head of the department of internal medicine at MH, was possibly the single most powerful man in the hospital. That the patient was responsible for a large chunk of the hospital's endowment obliged it to provide him with the most high-powered care possible. His attending wrote daily notes on his progress, and called his buddies, the heads of the other departments—

psychiatry, neurology, and the rest—to come and do consults on him.

Mr. Cloud was a small, old, bald man, used to getting what he wanted in life and taking orders from no one. The fact that he had been confined to a hospital room against his wishes for talking about suicide drove him absolutely crazy, and he refused to talk to anyone about wanting to kill himself.

Regardless, his doctors dutifully worked him up for suicidal ideation. His head was scrutinized by every possible method. Its structure was rudely probed with X rays and CAT scans. Its electrical activity was measured by sticking two million little tiny wires into his scalp to record an electroencephalogram. Its content was explored during endless psychiatric interviews, some of which were spent with the patient fuming in total silence.

I dropped into Mr. Cloud's room once a day to say hello. I enjoyed this enormously because all the people hanging around outside his door stopped whatever hushed conversations they were having and acted very deferential, saying, "Oh! Here comes Daddy's (Uncle's, Grandpa's, Mr. Cloud's) doctor to examine him. Let him through!" There were usually a few people hanging around inside his room, too, all looking at the patient with pleading gazes while he sat looking angry and bored.

I'd say, "Sorry, folks, I just need a few minutes with Mr. Cloud so you'll have to step out." I got a real kick out of how around 35 carats' of diamond and two or three grand of Italian silk would get on up and skedaddle just because some slightly greasy little kid wearing an M.D. tag told 'em to be on their way.

As I saw it, Mr. Cloud was just a little too old and a little too feeble for his own liking and he didn't feel like living anymore. He was bored and wanted to die. I had few feelings about this one way or the other. I was an intern wallowing up to my ass in other people's piss, vomit, blood, and shit, as well as my own whining self-pity, and didn't spend a whole lot of time thinking about him. I had absolutely nothing to gain by putting on a show of concern. No money, no time, no gratitude, and I was in no mood to behave selflessly. Even if I was vaguely interested in seeing the patient "improve," a vestige of my once so important desire to "help" people, I knew I had no realistic chance of influencing him. If the best brains MH had to offer couldn't budge him, what was I to do? I only asked once about what was bothering him.

He said, "I'm too old."

I told him suicide wasn't legal and he'd have to stay locked up until he gave up the idea. He appreciated my failure to put on an act about being deathly serious and concerned with what was wrong with him and adopted a half-interested sort of fatherlike approach to me and asked me questions about my life.

The major problem with Mr. Cloud's hospital stay was that he had too many doctors. What he needed was one single doc who was responsible for his case and his follow-up. Instead, he had a half-dozen docs who puffed up their chests, made grave declarations about the need for esoteric blood tests performed only at the Centers for Disease Control in Atlanta, and passed him off to each other like a hot potato. No one simply sat down and dealt with him.

Despite all of his high-powered docs, I had a fair amount of control over Mr. Cloud's hospitalization. As his intern, I wrote all of his orders. His attending and the consulting docs wrote what they wanted for the patient in their notes and, if I could decipher their scribbles, I made sure they got done. Technically, I also had the power to discharge the patient from the hospital, though doing so without permission from his attending would cause serious trouble. Nonetheless, it would be easy to do. I'd tell the hangers-on outside his room that I wanted Mr. Cloud to have one night of complete rest and solitude and to please leave and come back in the morning. Later in the evening I'd tell the desk clerk and the head nurse that I was discharging him, that the order was written, and that he was dressed and ready to go. With that he could simply walk out of the hospital. Although an underhanded way of doing it, designed to circumvent the private docs lurking about during the day, it would work just fine.

Mr. Cloud knew I had this power and begged me on a daily basis to get him out of the hospital. One day, in very serious tones, he said, "Now, listen to me, Joseph [he always used my first name], I will set you up for the rest of your life if you discharge me from this hospital. I give you my absolute word on it, I will set you up for the rest of your life."

The horrible part of this story is that I never took him up on this, but instead played the role of good intern.

I said, "Now Mr. Cloud, the doctors who are taking care of you are very concerned about you and you know I can't do that."

What crap! It would've been much more interesting to say, "Well, Mr. Cloud, ol' pal, just what exactly do you mean by 'set me up for the rest of my life'?" Every time I think about it now I get an anguished feeling of lost possibility.

Still, there was a hateful, heinous part of me that enjoyed the power I had over Mr. Cloud. Regardless of all his wealth and power, he couldn't buy off a little twenty-six-year-old kid who held him prisoner in the hospital. Not only that, but I could dangle the carrot before his eyes in the name of "good medical care." How amusing. How I loved internship.

Eventually all of Mr. Cloud's consultants got together and decided it was time to discharge him from the hospital. By this time I was so disconnected from the case that I had no idea whether he was still suicidal or not. I just wrote the discharge order and proceeded to the next patient. Several months later I learned that he finally got his wish. I guess he managed to pull the wool over the eyes of the best brains MH had to offer after all. Good thing I didn't let him buy himself out of the hospital because everyone would blame me, try to have me fired, take away my medical license, sue me, and the rest of it. Of course they'd be having a hell of a time scouring all the little tiny islands of the South Pacific trying to find me and my millions.

4

The Patient Even
Bellevue Didn't Want

Medical training as it exists today dates to 1910, when the Carnegie Foundation funded a report ("The Flexner Report") about medical education in the United States. Its author surveyed all of the medical schools in the country, finding widely varying levels of quality. The majority of schools were criticized as poorly disguised degree mills with little regard for the skills of the students they graduated, while those (such as Johns Hopkins and Harvard) that had university affiliations, extensive laboratory facilities, and ample patient populations were held as the ideal. "The Flexner Report" soon found its way into policy with the development of standard criteria for medical education. The next several decades saw a decline in both the number of medical schools and the number of doctors graduated.

The medical establishment argues, and not unreasonably so, that "The Flexner Report" and the system of formal and uniform accreditation of doctors that arose from it has resulted in a dramatic increase in the quality of medical practice in the United States. Although this is in large measure true, one of its effects has been a decrease in the practice of lay medicine. In the last century people in communities all over the nation were provided health care through an extensive network of lay nurses, doctors, healers, herbalists, surgeons, and midwives, who were widespread and unregulated. Most had learned their skills as apprentices. "The Flexner Report" ended much of this practice, criticizing it as bad medicine foisted on an unsuspecting public. One can't help wondering, however, to what extent its findings fit hand in glove with the desire of the medical establishment to reduce competition from lay medical practitioners and gain complete control of a lucrative profession.

Having completed college and successfully clawed his way into med school, the summa cum laude graduate is dumped back at the bottom of the heap as a beginning med student. In the first and second years of med school, he spends the vast majority of his time battling an avalanche of information, some two thousand years' worth of accumulated biomedical knowledge. The second two years are spent in clinical clerkships, where, agglutinated to resident/intern teams, the student is introduced to the catastrophe of residency and the distorted personalities he'll meet there.

Perhaps the strangest aspect of the entire process of becoming a doctor is its competitiveness. Competition, one-upmanship, outdoing one's colleagues, being the best and the brightest, is central to the process from high school right through residency and fellowship. Though it might be rationalized that this selects those best suited to reach the top of the profession, my experience showed that this is not true. What competition does is teach students in college and med school, and docs in residency, how best to be competitive, how to hone their skills in the traditional academic sense. Though most start the whole business because they really do want to help people, they soon learn that it is their ability to compete, rather than their love of humanity, that counts. The people who make it into medical school and then into the hot-shot residencies are the ones who get the best grades, not the ones who demonstrate the most compassion for their fellow man. Unfortunately, these skills are not the most important aspects of being a good doc. It is certainly necessary to be competent, but equally vital is that old, clichéd desire to help people, that the doc be a real human being and not just an academic overachiever.

Our teachings in college and medical school did not prepare us for what we encountered when we finally arrived on the Cloud Pavilion. What we yearned for, what we had been trained for in medical school, was a patient we could cure. The curable patient was the medical ideal. The curable patient was the one described in the medical journals. It wasn't even a total loss if the patient died, so long as we could point at something, a diseased organ, a killer X ray, an amazingly abnormal blood test, and say, "There it is! That's what we were after, and that's what we got (or missed)." And that was the kind of patient that was few and far between on the Cloud Pavilion.

Chronicity, incurability, "untunability," frustrated us. Instead of looking at these entities as something to deal with, to cope with, we'd learned to battle them. Chronically ill and terminal patients were rarely told, "Here are the facts and here are the possibilities for living the remainder of your life in comfort" and were all too often used as medical battlegrounds.

As I sat atop Uncle Melvin stuffing a tube into his nose, I never stopped once to say, "Well, Mel, is it enough already? Are you sick of being treated like a lab animal? Are you wondering how many more times you're going to get pneumonia and be tortured like this?" That

71

Mel couldn't answer was not the point. The point was that I repressed these thoughts and feelings and then wondered what was making me so anxious. I never wrote irate letters to the newspapers, or demanded of my seniors, my role models, "We're torturing these people. Please tell me why we are torturing these people!" My job was not to ask such questions. My job was to cure Mel's pneumonia and boot him back to the nursing home. No one ever bothered to inquire about my feelings or the patient's feelings on the subject. In medical school they said, "This is what pneumonia looks like and this is what you do about it." They never said, "By the way, one day you're going to be on call, and you're going to be torturing some old guy, and at some point you may even develop some feelings about it and here are our suggestions about how to cope with those feelings." We were simply told, "This is what pneumonia looks like, and this is how you cure it, and isn't that great!"

So, we did our job, we treated the pneumonia believing that this was the most important possible thing we could do; identify the lesion and attack. Then, after some time went by, after we'd tortured dozens of people in the name of medical care, we found that pneumonia was not really the biggest problem. We discovered that chronicity was the problem, incurable disease was the problem, hopes and dreams stifled by illness was the problem. And, because no one taught us how to cope with chronicity, or incurability, or hopes and dreams stifled by illness, we spent our time continually trying to cure the pneumonia and wondering why we were so unhappy. It should come as little surprise that we eventually reacted to this by ceasing to care. How could we care when it was so obvious that our actions had very little to do with the emotional and spiritual lives of our patients? Instead, we simply focused on getting rid of our patients as quickly as possible, and getting the hell out of the hospital.

But for the fact that it was incurable, AIDS might have been the best possible thing to have come along and stroke our egos. Here was a disease with meat, a disease that allowed us to point in awe at fascinating X rays or amazing blood tests. Here was a disease that struck the young and vital instead of the old and feeble. Here was a disease, by God, that we could cure! One where we could "cure the pneumonia" and where this was, after all, the most important thing to be done for the patient.

The only problem was that we couldn't cure it. It became the chronic, progressive, incurable, debilitating disease of the young. Just what we needed. Sure, we could treat at least some of its esoteric sequelae. The patient didn't actually die of the underlying immune disorder caused by the virus (human immunodeficiency virus, or HIV), he died of the so-called opportunistic infections, bizarre viral pneumonias, and fungal infestations of the central nervous system that resulted from this immune deficiency. We treated these infections over and over and over again, but could do nothing about their cause, nothing to fix the patients' immune systems, just like we could add or subtract a liter from Mr. Kram without being able to fix his heart.

And, for many of the AIDS patients we couldn't even treat the opportunistic infections. For those with viral pneumonias we were totally powerless. We were thrown back to the preantibiotic era, when doctors could only take X ray after X ray, and watch the pneumonia get bigger and bigger until the patient finally died of asphyxiation. In fact, it was worse than bacterial pneumonias in the preantibiotic days because, back then, the pneumonia sometimes resolved spontaneously. However, when an AIDS patient got a herpetic pneumonia he was a dead man. There was no possibility for a spontaneous cure.

We simply tuned up the oxygen until it was running full tilt and there was no healthy lung left to absorb it and the patient died.

I attended to many AIDS patients during my medical training. Most were admitted not to Cloud, but to New York General Hospital, Manhattan Hospital's sister institution. While Manhattan Hospital was a private, not-for-profit institution (ha, ha, ha), NYG was a city hospital. The medical service at Manhattan Hospital admitted mostly older patients of private docs, and NYG handled younger, poorer people who walked into the emergency room off the street.

None of the patients at NYG had private docs, and were cared for by resident/intern teams in consultation with their team attendings. We called the hospital "W-NNN-Y-G," in parody of a popular radio announcer who pronounced his radio station "W-NNN-B-C."

Junkies made up a good 25-30 percent of the admissions at NYG. Because of AIDS, and because of the risk of AIDS created by intravenous drug abuse, we admitted virtually every junkie who came into the emergency room with a fever as "rule-out AIDS."

By virtue of the very fact that they are junkies, junkies have received relatively little press in the whole AIDS issue. Homosexual men, on the other hand, a "community" to start with, have organized themselves. They have formed the Gay Men's Health Crisis and other intrinsic organizations whose goal is to educate gay men about, and therefore prevent, the spread of AIDS. They have gained political clout. They have pressed legislation. And, as recent statistical data demonstrating a decline in the spread of new HIV virus infection among homosexual men has shown, they have been quite successful.

Junkies, on the other hand, do not exist as a "community." The very consuming nature of their behavior, and the fact of its illegality, prevents the formation of an "Intravenous Drug Abusers' Health Crisis." Drug abuse treatment programs and small outreach projects exist; unfortunately, potential junkie clients outnumber available treatment slots by about 500 to 1. Junkies are virtually wholly dependent on the kindness of strangers to rescue them from their dilemma. And, for the vast majority, strangers have not been very kind.

Such shabby treatment is a pity, a damn shame, because not only does it reflect the callousness of society, but it is the major factor that puts society at risk for the further spread of AIDS, its spread into the heterosexual population. Gay men do not represent an enormous threat to heterosexuals because, for the most part, gay men do not engage in heterosexual relations. Junkies, on the other hand, do have sex with women, and it is precisely at this point that a major "vector" of the disease into the heterosexual population is found. In fact, the glimmers of attention that have appeared in the last year or so regarding evidence of continued, atrociously high rates of spread of the virus among junkies has probably been motivated by this very concern, rather than by any real worry for the junkies themselves.

Realistically, however, those at greatest risk are poor women, the sexual partners of male junkies. The poor areas of New York, those areas where junkies live, and where women have sex with these men (in many cases not knowing that their partners are abusing drugs) are being decimated by AIDS. It is not unusual for an entire family to be destroyed, for the father to pass it off to the mother, and the mother to a fetus who later becomes a child with AIDS. I have seen more than one single woman sitting alone in the emergency room awaiting admission for treatment of her first AIDS-related infection, single only because her husband and child were already dead. Most such single women were under the age of thirty.

In addition to working on Cloud, I spent a good portion of my internship year working on the medical wards of NYG, where I treated many junkies. It was here that I had the most exposure to AIDS though I saw the occasional AIDS patient when I was an intern on Cloud, too.

One such AIDS patient was a transvestite hooker junkie named Miss Davis. Miss Davis hadn't had a sex change operation but dressed like a woman and preferred to be considered a woman. I acceded to his preference. I asked him what he wanted to be called and he said "Miss Davis," so that's what I called him, and whenever I spoke to someone else about him in his presence, like at morning rounds, I used the word "she."

Miss Davis was sick as a dog with AIDS. She'd originally presented herself at Bellevue Hospital's emergency room (ER), feverish and coughing up a storm. Unfortunately, all the beds in Bellevue were full, so the medical admitting resident (MAR), the third-year medical resident in charge of approving and assigning admissions, called NYG to request a transfer. The call was received by the MAR at NYG, who listened carefully to the patient's description and decided that she was too sick to be transferred, even though NYG had available beds. He said he didn't want to risk the patient tubing in the ambulance and told the MAR at Bellevue he'd have to treat her in his ER until one of his own beds became available.

It should come as little surprise that managing the patient in this manner had little to do with her own welfare. The MAR's primary job was not to ensure that sick people got admitted to the hospital, as might be thought, but to protect the housestaff on call from being overworked by too many admissions. Also, by refusing the transfer, the MAR protected himself from any screwup that might occur while the patient was en route, a period for which he was legally responsible.

Miss Davis showed up at NYG about an hour later in a cab. All the residents on call at Bellevue had chipped in to provide the fare and get her the hell out of their hospital. They told her they had no room and offered her the money to get to NYG if she'd sign a paper certifying that she'd refused treatment at Bellevue. This was called signing out, and protected the hospital if the patient crumped after leaving. In this way the residents used the money not only to get rid of the patient, but as a bribe to protect themselves. A medical maxim: "CYA," or "cover your ass." If the MAR at NYG called to complain they could say, "Hey, look, the patient signed out and we have the papers here to prove it. At least we had the decency to give her cab fare to get to another hospital." Miss Davis was a medical hot potato, the patient even Bellevue didn't want.

I was working as an intern on the medical floors at NYG and admitted Miss Davis to my team. I liked her. She was quiet, civil, polite, and didn't scream obscenities at random passersby like most of the junkies. Her sexual achievements as a hooker were astounding. I asked her roughly how many sexual encounters she'd had, rounding off to the nearest ten, and she said, "Oh, around five or ten thousand." Perhaps it was naïveté, but I was fantastically impressed by that. I don't think she enjoyed her lifestyle. It was simply necessary to support her drug habit. Junkies do strange things.

One of the strange things that Miss Davis did was called "skin popping." This truly horrible habit, in which the junkie sticks the needle under the skin and shoots in the junk, is practiced by those whose veins (the usual route of administration for junk) have scarred over before they die or quit. The syringes and needles used by junkies are notoriously unclean, absolutely filthy, and cause frequent infections. Large open sores and areas of thick scar-

77

ring abound, ruining even the prettiest of physiques.

I completely forgot to ask Miss Davis about skin popping, which she'd been doing on her legs for a long time. She also didn't volunteer telling me about it. After I finished taking her history I did a physical exam and received quite a shock. I threw back the bedsheets to check her feet for swelling (part of a routine exam) and came damn close to tossing my cookies right on the spot. There was little skin remaining on her legs, which were covered with open sores and islands of thick, ragged scar tissue. There were even areas of bone showing. It was really awful.

I may be upset by something, but I can keep my cool if I at least know it's coming. Had someone said, "Listen, you should brace yourself before you look at her legs," I would have been okay. I took a deep breath to cover up my shock and excused myself from the room to collect myself.

Later I called the surgeons to have a look and suggest how to deal with her legs. I think one or two of them almost lost their cookies, too.

Miss Davis definitely was an oddball. People who defend the rights of transvestites, hookers, and junkies may take offense at that, but it was true. Many of the doctors at NYG had problems with their attitudes about Miss Davis and it showed in the way they treated her. Perhaps the fact that she was black, a transvestite, a hooker, a junkie, and had disgusting legs made them think that she had some kind of super-AIDS. Most of the consultants who came to see her gloved, gowned, and wore masks whenever they went into the room. It was still early on in terms of understanding AIDS and though it seemed clear that the sole source of risk lay in the exchange of body fluids, people were still jittery. I couldn't blame the non-medical staff but was annoyed by paranoia in doctors. They were supposed to know better. If they didn't want to deal with people who were dangerously sick they were working in the wrong damn place.

A great deal of AIDS paranoia persists today, years after this episode. More and more groups of docs, particularly surgeons, are coming out with statements declaring that they will forthwith refuse to treat AIDS patients. Their rationale is that the risk of infection is too great, that the chance of exposure to the blood of AIDS patients is too high. I wonder what happened to the oath that such docs took when they became M.D.'s. What they might have done fifty years ago when mere presence in the room of a patient with any of a number of infectious diseases was enough to risk possibly fatal infection, when simply being in a country suffering an outbreak of plague was risking death. Don't these folks know that AIDS is the first in an endless series of deadly epidemics that can be controlled by behavior alone? Sexually, don't be promiscuous. Recreationally, don't shoot up. And, in the operating room, cover precious surgeons from head to foot, as though they were about to take a walk in space, so they don't risk exposure to the deadly virus.

Those who consider this a load of self-righteous crap and claim that accidents just can't be avoided are right. Risk is part of the job, and those who want complete safety should consider working elsewhere.

I sat down with Miss Davis and told her, frankly speaking, that many of the doctors would treat her like she was a leper or had the plague and she shouldn't take it personally. She didn't blink during this speech. She'd probably heard it so many times before that it was old hat and was just being polite. I half expected her to yawn and say, "You naïve child, if you think I don't know they believe I'm from Mars, you've got another think coming."

Another of Miss Davis's odd traits was her willingness to let doctors do anything and everything to her they wanted without ever putting up a fuss. Shortly after she was admitted, for example, we had to put a great big IV (a central line) into her neck because all of the veins on her arms were scarred over and unusable. When I sat down to explain the procedure and get her written consent, I expected her to put up an enormous stink, a reasonable reaction to the suggestion of sticking a gigantic, pencil-sized needle into someone's neck. When I finished the explanation she said, "Okay," and didn't ask any questions at all.

She said the same thing when I told her she needed bronchoscopy. Bronchoscopy would entail sticking a big fiberoptic tube into her mouth and then down into her windpipe and right down into her lungs. Once it was in the lungs the pulmonologists (lung docs) would peer around by looking in the part of the tube sticking out of her mouth. Using a little claw on the end of the tube, they'd tear off a little piece of lung to subject to tests. Bronchoscopy is right out of *Fantastic Voyage*.

Peering around in someone's lungs and tearing off little pieces for testing can be useful if a patient has some form of fancy or esoteric pneumonia. This was the case with Miss Davis. I told her all of this and she said, "Okay." It was as though she had no idea why she was in the hospital but was perfectly content to hang out and let the occasional strange white man in a long white coat come into her room and ram some sort of tube into her, mumbling some gibberish to other white men in long white coats.

Perhaps Miss Davis's willingness to consent to just about anything was merely a carryover from her occupation. Whatever the reason, it was no help in getting the consultants to deal with her. AIDS paranoia lurked everywhere. The lung docs covered up their fear by complaining about the long and arduous task of cleaning their very expensive lung-peering tubes, which would be covered with AIDS germs. As AIDS was slated to be the disease of the decade, and possibly the century, and since the lung docs were seeing two or three new AIDS patients a day, I wondered if the hospital would spring for a set of bronchoscopes to be used on queers and junkies only. Until that day came, I was told, they'd be "scoping" only those AIDS patients who were true diagnostic dilemmas. I scratched my head and asked what, in that case, was I supposed to treat him for. Everything, they said.

I got on the phone to speak to the bug doc (the infectious disease consultant) and asked what medications to use to treat everything. The bug doc suggested nafcillin, gentamycin, vancomycin, trimethoprim, sulfamethoxazole, ethambutol, PAS, rifampin, triple sulfa, and amphotericin (also known as amphoterrible). It was hoped that this incredibly fearsome combination, if it didn't kill the patient first, would kill every microorganism known to man, except, of course, the virus that had caused the AIDS to start with.

I later realized that treating for everything meant that there'd never be a diagnostic dilemma for the lung docs. They'd say, "Well, we don't need to scope the patient because you're treating for every possible cause of pneumonia anyway, so we can't find anything useful." Nice going, I thought, very well done. Nobody wanted to get near the AIDS patients so we'd cover 'em with shotgun blasts until they either got better or died.

As it turned out, Miss Davis did die. She developed a red-alert lab value that was missed because the doc taking care of her at the time was too exhausted to see straight. I didn't feel so bad about her death because I knew for certain that this particular doctor had nothing against AIDS patients.

I had a strange feeling that as Miss Davis's blood pressure was dropping and people were running around making noise and poking her with needles and looking frantic, she figured it was all just another part of the whole act. I could see her, even as she lay stone dead, her eyes wide

81

open while people were pumping on her chest, as though to say, "Well, you just go right on ahead with whatever you want to do. It's okay with me."

I went to Miss Davis's autopsy wondering if it would be a learning experience or would leave a deep scar in my emotional psyche. Autopsies are exceedingly bizarre to start with and because I knew the subject, this one would be all the more strange. As I watched her get hacked apart I felt sad, upset, and fascinated all at the same time.

Incredibly, the pathologist was an elderly man with a German accent wearing a bow tie and round wire-frame glasses. He pointed to little squiggly black lines all over the surface of Miss Davis's disemboweled lungs and said, "Unt, do you know vhat zeez are?"

"Carbon deposits," I replied. "From breathing city air."

"Ja, ja, very goot," he said. "Unt do you know vy zeez lungs are zo boggy unt hev zeez leetle dots?" The lungs had the consistency of a soaking-wet sponge. Healthy lungs would have the consistency of a fairly well wrung-out sponge. They had little red dots all over them, as though a Hollywood makeup artist were trying to give them the appearance of having the measles.

I said, "Tuberculosis?" and he ejaculated, "Ja! Very goot!" I left feeling somehow satisfied that the story had a neat and clean ending and eventually I forgot all about Miss Davis.

I should add that a number of years have passed since I met Miss Davis, and the public health bureaucracy has finally dragged its ever slothful eye to a comprehensive view of the AIDS crisis. There has even been recognition of the critical steps that must be taken to arrest the spread of the disease among poverty-stricken drug abusers. Congress has set aside money to expand the availability of treatment for addiction, as well as for programs designed to reach the junkie in the street. True, a billion dollars probably won't do the job, especially after all the politicians take their dip, but it's a start.

5

Smoking and Booze

Like lemmings rushing off the edge of a cliff, Americans drink, smoke, inject, ingest, and inflict violence on themselves and others in a manner so fast and furious that the medical head spins. Having conquered the plagues such as cholera and tuberculosis that once decimated entire populations, it seems that Americans now feel obligated to discover new, exciting, and creative ways to destroy themselves.

We have done a terrific job. As a nation we have created epidemics of heart disease, liver disease, lung disease, and cancer in proportions never before seen. We have created new and bizarre malignancies that never before existed. And, amazingly, we are fully aware of the causes of these epidemics, fully aware that we have brought them upon ourselves, fully aware that they are preventable. Yet, both as a society and as individuals we have done little or nothing to stop them.

Plainly put, it is poison that kills Americans. Poison in the air, poison in the water, poison in food, and, of course, the poisons we use intentionally, which result in our chemical dependencies. We are a nation in love with poison.

The list of favorite poisons is topped by cigarettes and alcohol. They are the deadliest poisons of all, accounting for more death in the United States than any other entity. The other "recreational drugs" kill but a mere fraction of the number slaughtered yearly by cigarettes and booze. Regardless, the list continues and is long and impressive. There are, for example, cocaine and heroin, two smash hits among the popular press. There are sundry sedatives such as Valium, Librium, and the barbiturates, and other drugs currently less in vogue, LSD and its hallucinogenic cousins, stimulants such as amphetamines, and less classifiable drugs such as the famed "angel dust" (phencyclidine), a drug once described to me as "horse tranquilizer," that falls somewhere between the class of hallucinogen and common gasoline additive. There are the alcohol substitutes, Sterno, antifreeze (ethylene glycol), turpentine, and wood alcohol (methanol). But, at the top, towering way above all the rest, there are cigarettes and booze.

Cigarette smoking alone is without question the single greatest cause of preventable mortality in the United States. Translated, cigarettes kill legions of people who wouldn't die if they didn't smoke, a statement that is supported by absolutely gargantuan statistical figures. The October 30, 1987, issue of *Mortality and Morbidity Weekly Report* (or MMWR), a charming publication put out by the Massachusetts Medical Society, attributed 200,000 deaths in 1980 directly to smoking, and over 300,000 in 1982. Smoking kills more Americans than anything else, period. It's killed more people than World War II, Korea, and Vietnam, more people than car accidents and enraged lovers, more people than heroin and cocaine, AIDS, barbiturates, Sterno, PCP, and LSD. It has killed more people than all of these factors *combined*. It causes cancer of the lips, oral cavity, neck, larynx, trachea, and lungs, and is the single greatest causative factor in all other forms of cancer. It causes emphysema and myriad other lung diseases. It causes heart attacks, heart failure, and stroke.

85

Interestingly, these entities comprise the plagues of modern Western society, and are the primary causes of what the MMWR calls "years of potential life lost before age 65." The moderate to heavy smoker is almost guaranteed to succumb to one of them. Nonsmokers die of similar causes, but live a good fifteen to twenty years longer than their smoking counterparts. Obesity and its consequences (particularly diabetes), polluted air, water, and food, violence, car accidents, the sequelae of alcoholism, and diseases of childhood account for virtually all of the rest of premature death in America.

Despite all of this, Americans are ferocious smokers, seeming unable to quit. One of my preceptors in medical school was a lung doc who said that smoking was perhaps the hardest addiction to quit, harder than drugs, alcohol, or overeating. He was a VA (Veteran's Administration) hospital doc and loved to cite as evidence for this the old hard-core vet smokers who were trached at the VA and could be seen rolling around the hallways in wheelchairs smoking Luckies and Camels through the holes in their necks.

A trach (medical slang for tracheostomy) is a hole drilled in a patient's neck right into his windpipe. Trachs are often done to people who have big-time neck surgery for messy throat tumors and no longer have the regular passages to breathe through. Ironically, people who smoked through their trachs were often trached for a problem related to smoking. Also, the act of smoking through a hole in the neck looked really strange. Some of the guys had special boxes they'd press up against their necks to create an artificial voice. The boxes made a weird twangy sound like a Jew's harp. A group of men in their fifties and sixties, their forearms and chests covered with graying hair and smudged tattoos, could be seen sitting in a cloud of smoke in the hallway, each using one hand to hold the box and talk and the other to smoke through his trach. A strange scene.

Battling with cigarettes for the title of most deadly legal recreational drug in the United States is alcohol. In addition to its direct physical effects on the body, alcohol is responsible for, or associated with, more than 50 percent of crime and violent death (including somewhere around 80 or 90 percent of car accidents) in the country. Alcohol's effects on the body alone are staggering. There isn't an organ system in the body that can't be poisoned by too much booze. Offhand, I can think of alcoholic fatty liver, alcoholic hepatitis, portal hypertension and ascites, cirrhosis of the liver, hepatic encephalopathy, gastritis, peptic ulcer disease, acute and chronic pancreatitis, esophageal varices, gastrointestinal bleeding, malnutrition, a variety of vitamin deficiencies, peripheral polyneuropathies, and Wernicke Korsakoff syndrome. Those are actual pathologic entities (a "pathologic entity" is a disease that can be identified by the actual changes it causes in an organ that can be seen under the microscope) and don't include the withdrawal syndromes: tremulousness, delirium tremens (DTs), alcoholic hallucinosis, seizures ("rum fits"), and death, the things people do to themselves and others when they are drunk, and the social and economic cost of being an alcoholic.

Not much fun. Of all the ways to kill oneself, death by alcohol is among the messiest and most painful. It is a process that is long and involved and, unless the alcoholic has the decency to die at home or in the street, one that generates an enormous amount of work for the intern on call.

Death by alcohol usually involves the consequences of cirrhosis of the liver. Cirrhosis is a complex process that causes both inflammation and scarring of the liver, and, unless alcohol abuse stops, eventual liver failure (so-called end-stage liver disease). A brief description of both liver anatomy and physiology will help put the plight of the unfortunate big-time alcoholic in better perspective.

The liver is an organ known vaguely to most as a large, brown, crescent-shaped blob of Jell-O-like consistency located somewhere within the abdominal cavity. This is exactly what it is, and here it performs functions critical to life. Its duties begin with the portal vein, a large blood vessel located on the right side of the abdominal cavity that collects blood from the intestines, fresh and bloated with fats, protein, carbohydrates, vitamins, minerals, and sundry food additives absorbed from digested food. The portal vein leads right into the liver, where it branches into a zillion tiny blood vessels that distribute the blood throughout the substance of the organ. Here the blood is in a sense filtered, and toxic substances are removed, metabolized, and rendered harmless.

All food, even health freak food, 100 percent natural and free of additives, contains toxins. Ammonia, a natural by-product of protein, is one such toxin cleared by the liver. Further, a large number of drugs are removed from the blood and inactivated in this manner. Doses of such drugs must be lowered in people suffering from diminished liver function.

The liver is the department of immigration and customs for the new arrivals from the intestines, screening the blood for contraband and illegal substances. Once it has made its way through the liver, blood proceeds to the inferior vena cava, the big vein that leads all the blood from the lower half of the body to the heart. As I've explained, the heart then reoxygenates the blood with a quick trip to the lungs and sends it back off to the tissues of the body to deliver its load of oxygen and nutrients.

Not absolutely all of the blood from the portal vein goes

through the liver. A few very small blood vessels bypass it altogether and enter the inferior vena cava directly, carrying small amounts of illicit, unscreened materials directly into the general circulation. In the healthy individual, this volume of blood is very small, and its contribution of unscreened toxins inconsequential.

Ethanol, the ever popular molecule found drifting in varying proportions in cooked hops, bitters, grape extracts, malts, or any number of other natural and artificial flavorings, is directly toxic to the liver. With each drink, both the "social drinker" and the big-time boozer damage their livers. Just one evening of serious boozing causes damage significant enough to be seen with the naked eye. Thus, when the social drinker ties on a good one and then kills himself in a car accident, the pathologist (autopsy doc) may note a certain swelling and bogginess in his liver, the changes of "fatty liver." If, on the other hand, the drinker survives the evening, awakens the next day with a roaring headache, swears off the grape forever, and does no drinking for several days, the liver repairs itself completely, fully restoring its normal anatomy.

The alcoholic gives his liver no such respite. Under a constant ethanol barrage, it is constantly sick. With repeated insults, it runs the pathologic gamut from fatty liver to alcoholic hepatitis, a condition in which it is angry, inflamed, enlarged, and tender, to cirrhosis. Each insult results in the development of a small area of scarred, dead tissue. Given time, the areas of scarring coalesce into larger such cirrhotic areas. Eventually, the scarred portion of the liver grows large enough that both its function and the nature of blood flow through the portal vein are affected.

Portal blood, on reaching the liver, finds burnt-out, boarded-up customs counters where there used to be gleaming, spotlessly kept, and smoothly functioning immigration facilities. Thousands and thousands of new arrivals are backed up at passport control and the portal vein becomes swollen with blood clamoring to enter the general circulation through the vena cava. Eventually, the pressure within it becomes so high that fluid from the blood begins to leak and weep out through its walls just as it had in the wayward, leaking blood vessels in Mr. Kram's soggy, gasping lungs. Because the portal vein is located in the abdominal cavity, the leaking fluid begins to accumulate around the belly and intestines. Before he knows it, the boozer develops a big, fat, fluid-filled abdomen that isn't very sexy at all.

Formerly law-abiding blood that would have been ushered directly through the liver now seeks other ways into the inferior vena cava. Like the narrow portions of the Rio Grande during the dry season, the little side vessels that bypass the liver develop sudden popularity. One of these is a network of feathery blood vessels that wind around the esophagus near its connection to the stomach and then enter the inferior vena cava. In people with cirrhosis the pressure of blood diverted away from the liver causes this formerly feathery net of blood vessels to become big and bloated. This becomes a problem by virtue of its tendency to bleed into the esophagus, causing the alcoholic to vomit blood.

In addition, the blood that bypasses the liver is totally unscreened, the toxins it carries flow freely into the inferior vena cava, like raw sewage from New York City being dumped directly into the Hudson River. Because the function of the liver itself is diminished, even the blood that is processed carries poisons into the general circulation. A number of these toxins, especially ammonia, have the effect of making the drinker go crazy, just like a verifiable crazy person, a condition called hepatic encephalopathy.

The big-time chronic alcoholic with big-time cirrhosis lies in bed, his gigantic, bloated, fluid-filled belly and malnourished, spindly arms and legs giving him the appearance of an enormous bedridden basketball. This, combined with an episode of vomiting blood and an ammonia-crazed mind, makes the drinker a pretty damn sorry sight.

There was a terrific Oriental intern at Manhattan Hospital who was on call one night taking care of a twenty-eight-year-old boozer with a major case of cirrhosis. After some very serious boozing, the patient had finally realized there was a good chance he would die and was scared shitless. Because he couldn't eat he was literally shitless, too. Though everyone knew he was headed for Cloud 9 he'd told his doctors that he wanted them to do everything possible for him. I saw him several times because he shared a room with one of my patients. I remember being a little (but not very) surprised by his age, and impressed by his big, pregnant-looking bellyful of portal vein juice. His hair was thinned out and downy-looking, and because he'd been in the hospital for a while he had an almost full downy beard. This did not belie his frightened baby face, or his glaring, fantastically bright, predeath eyes.

In his most recent binge of drinking the patient had finally blown out the last remaining piece of functioning liver in his body. He lay in bed as this last chunk flared up, white-hot and bright like the last match of a book set on fire, and then settled to smolder and finally die. As part and parcel of cirrhosis, he was suffering a terrible case of a bleeding esophagus. One night he began to bleed like there was no tomorrow, which in his case proved true. The formerly feathery but now bloated blood vessels around his esophagus (known medically as esophageal varices) bled furiously and unabated, pouring literally liters of blood into his esophagus and stomach, which he'd then vomit up all over his bedsheets. A very messy scene.

The Oriental resident told me, "He start vomiting up all his blood about nine o'clock."

I said, "So, what'd you do?"

He replied, "I get blood from blood bank and try to replace all the blood he throw up."

I asked him if he considered putting a tube into the patient's stomach where all the blood was and putting the other end into a vein, kind of recirculate the same blood, and he said, "Hey, I didn't think of that, but good idea for future reference."

Then I asked him, "So, what happened?"

He replied, "He bleed and bleed and bleed and keep pulling out IV from thrashing around in bed."

I said, "Why was he thrashing around in bed?" and he said, "Because he have big-time case of hepatic encephalopathy and go completely crazy."

I asked, "So what wound up happening?"

The resident replied, "I tie him down so he can't pull out IV anymore and he keep bleeding and throwing up blood and finally die at about eight in the morning without letting me sleep at all."

What an ungrateful, selfish bastard.

Almost as exciting, equally dangerous, and as much a pain in the ass to treat as a good, brisk vericeal bleeder is an alcoholic suffering from delirium tremens. DTs are what happens when the serious drinker stops drinking. They are the culminating event in the process of withdrawal from alcohol, and can happen anytime from one to four days after a boozer gives up booze. The alcoholic suffering delirium tremens is very agitated, jittery, and does and sees weird things. The phrase "delirium tremens" describes this state quite well with its heavy medicalesque tones. Delirium is an excited mental state marked by hallucinations and illusions, and tremens are jitters. People with DTs get so agitated and weird that they do things that are destructive to themselves, like jump out of windows, or to others, like attack them in a mad frenzy. Also, people with DTs sometimes get so jittery they develop seizures.

The treatment for this condition is sedation, which calms the tremors and helps prevent seizures. Sedation, in fact, has the same effect in DTs as would a good stiff drink. When a boozer wakes up in the morning feeling jittery and agitated he goes to a bar (or the kitchen cupboard) for a drink more to relieve the jitters than for pleasure. Most addicts continue their habit not primarily because the poison continues to feel good, but because staying off is too painful.

Modern "detox" programs get people off drugs or booze by substituting another substance and gradually decreasing the dose to minimize withdrawal symptoms. Opiate addicts are given methadone and boozers are given sedatives. Drinkers admitted for detox are placed on Valium, Librium, phenobarbital, or any other sedative except booze and slowly tapered down until they are free of both drugs and alcohol. Decreasing doses of booze could probably also be used to bring a drinker through the DTs to a state of dryness, though I don't know the details of this possibility. I assume we use sedation to avoid alcohol's toxic effects on the liver as well as to modify drinking behavior.

Rather than going completely bananas and seizing, the detoxing drinker goes through a relatively calm two- to four-day period of pink elephants, whispering voices, mysterious insects, bizarre dreams, and generalized low-grade craziness until things start to get a little more lucid and normal.

The pink elephants, voices, and insects result from auditory and visual hallucinations, and illusions. A hallucination is completely fabricated by the mind, for example the patient's belief that he is having a conversation with a ghost while he is tied into bed. Pink elephants and whispering voices fall into the category of hallucinations. Illusions, which are usually visual, involve seeing something and imagining it to be something else. A curtain blowing in the wind becomes a shadowy burglar climbing in the window. A stain on the wall is a cockroach.

People who are in the process of having hallucinations and illusions believe they are very real. I've had the experience of joining a group conversation between a patient and his long-dead parents. The patient, referring to a comment made by a phantom parent, asked me several times whether I agreed. I had to apologize for continually asking him to repeat the comment. Eventually he saw a bug on the wall, forgot his parents, and began to scream, "Kill it! Kill it!" A very strange scene.

Alcoholics detox to freedom from drugs much more quickly than heroin addicts. The boozer is clean of booze in a few days while the heroin addict may remain on an opiate, methadone, for years, even decades. Drug freedom, however, is just the beginning for the reformed drinker. Alcoholics Anonymous, the famed support group for drinkers, is the next critical step in the process. I've yet to meet a boozer who managed to stay dry without the help of AA. Luckily for drinkers, the methods of AA are tried-and-true, unlike the record of most methadone centers. Though several principles underlie the AA program, the foremost is that each alcoholic rely on and be relied on by other reformed drinkers. AA is a brilliant organization and provides a brilliant example of approaching a social problem socially, rather than applying Band-Aids with science and medicine.

I helped care for an alcoholic patient while I was an intern on the surgical service at NYG, during the second half of the internship year. The patient went into florid DTs shortly after having surgery for a ruptured, infected

94

pancreatic pseudocyst. This condition, which a surgeon would call an "intra-abdominal catastrophe," was also a complication of his booze habit.

The pancreas, like the liver, suffers under the effect of alcohol, running the gamut from mild inflammation to catastrophic disease. In the initial stage, pancreatitis, the organ is inflamed, red, tender, and swollen, like the liver during a bout of alcoholic hepatitis. Normally, the pancreas produces digestive enzymes that are secreted into the intestines to break down food. As pancreatitis progresses, the organ actually begins to digest itself. In extreme cases it gets swollen like a big melon; the center is hollow and filled with a sloppy soup of the organ's own digested tissue, an entity known as a pancreatic pseudocyst. Given enough time, the soup gets infected; given more time the infected pseudocyst ruptures and a toxic soup of bacteria and caustic enzymes sloshes into the entire abdominal cavity, eating up and infecting everything in sight. A patient who has a pancreatic pseudocyst has big trouble; one who has an infected, ruptured pseudocyst has very big, life-threatening trouble, an intra-abdominal catastrophe.

Such patients must be taken to the OR and sheared open from the rib cage to the pelvis (a surgeon would say "from stem to stern") for a major cleaning and overhaul. After attempting to drain off the caustic slop from around the intestines, stomach, and other abdominal viscera, a task that might well be accomplished with a big soup ladle, the surgeon rinses the abdomen with a few dozen liters of sterile saline solution and leaves the wound wide open, flapping in the breeze. A rubber tube is put into the pseudocyst so that any further infected pancreatic muck produced will drain outside the abdomen. When the infection is cured, a task achieved by several times daily washing and rinsing the pancreas through the rubber tube in combination with several thousand dollars' worth of esoteric antibiotics, the patient is taken back to the OR to be sewed closed again.

Naturally, a patient with an open belly is a bad candidate for walking around the hospital corridors if his guts are to be prevented from dropping out onto the freshly waxed floor. It's a hell of a job getting someone from the housekeeping department to come and rewax them. This is the kind of patient for whom the "Activities" portion of the admitting orders would read "Strict bedrest" (not even allowing "Bathroom privileges").

Mr. Mendez had just gotten back from the OR and just gone into DTs when I first met him. He had a big open wound in his abdomen, allowing me to peer right down into his shiny, freshly drained, red pseudocyst. The deranged organ was infected with pseudomonas, a vicious and difficult-to-kill bug that, strangely, is not at all unpleasant smelling. One of the first things I noted on peering into the patient's infected belly was a pleasant scent, as though there were an open bottle of rosewater in his room.

Mr. Mendez was not being at all cooperative with our efforts to attend him properly. Although he was tied into his intensive care unit bed and had several surgical interns sitting on his chest, he persisted in squirming about and attempting to sit up in order to talk to friends whom he imagined to be in the room with him. He'd yell, "Rico! Carlos!" and babble in Spanish in a hurt tone of voice as though to impart to the people restraining him that he should simply be left in peace. One of the housestaff had draped a sterile towel over the surgical wound in his abdomen. Every time he started to struggle and tense his belly muscles, the housestaff fellow leaned on the towel with both hands to prevent him from squeezing his bowels out of the wound. Disemboweling, or eviscerating, himself is what a surgeon would call it.

By virtue of struggling, Mr. Mendez had succeeded in pulling out his IV and I was involved with a few other interns in trying to put in a new one. After several attempts I managed to get a catheter into a blood vessel, but on attaching the catheter to the IV bag, blood rushed up the tubing into the bag. This meant I had cannulated the radial artery by accident, pretty poor form, so I had to pull the line out and try again. Mr. Mendez looked particularly hurt when I resumed the stabbing.

At NYG pentobarbital was the standard drug for use in treating DTs. The standard dose was 100 milligrams every four hours. In intern's slang this was known as "600 hertz" since the total daily dose was 600 mg.

Our use of pentobarb was dictated by Dr. Big, the president of the hospital, who was known both for strong patient advocacy and vicious treatment of the housestaff. Interns feared having a patient become the subject of weekly teaching conferences chaired by Dr. Big, knowing they would be bloodied by his relentless onslaughts, charges of "idiocy," "having gone to medical school at Auschwitz," and the like, his gentle means of expressing an absolutely vicious intolerance of any form of weakness, incompetence, or error on the part of the housestaff. Most of the interns regarded him with a mix of respect, anger, and fear. My feelings were also mixed; I understood his point, but I wasn't sure that terrorism was an effective means of producing humane and skilled physicians.

Dr. Big insisted on the use of pentobarb because he believed that the frequent dosing schedule meant a close eye would be kept on the patient. When people who'd worked at NYG treated DTs elsewhere they'd insist on using any sedative other than pentobarb, not because of any advantage for the patients, but because there wasn't a thing Dr. Big could say or do about it.

I knew only one doc who ever dared to face up to Dr. Big. She was a young woman named Dolores, an extraordinarily dedicated doc who approached everything in life with the bizarre assumption that human beings were entitled to be treated as human beings. She dealt with everyone in the exact same fashion, straightforward and honest, from the slimiest junkie to the most offensive attending doc.

We were working together on the medical floors at NYG and had the task one week of presenting a case at Dr. Big's teaching conference. Dr. Big, in his usual form, was attempting to rip to shreds everything my partner or I had to say about the case. Finally, he asked Dolores a particularly esoteric question, the kind that only a specialist might be able to answer, and when she was unable to reply, demanded to know, "What kind of asshole would have the gall to call himself doctor and not know the answer to that question?"

Dolores gazed at his reddening face for a few moments, bearing an expression of almost motherly concern, and finally replied, "Well, Dr. Big, I'm sure there are many of us here in this room who don't know the answer to that question. Perhaps we could all learn a valuable point if you were to give it to us, so please do." There was absolutely no sarcasm in her voice. She sat down, folded her hands in her lap, and awaited his answer. The other residents in the room sat in dumbfounded silence. Dr. Big, steaming visibly, had no choice but to answer the question. It was a wonderful moment.

In treating drunks, care had to be taken with dosage in order to ensure that the patient was neither under nor oversedated. Mr. Mendez was grossly undersedated. After waking up from surgery, he'd been given 100 mg of pentobarb, which absolutely hadn't touched him. The functioning portions of alcoholics' livers are tremendously churned up metabolically because of all the booze they process, and can break down other drugs incredibly quickly. This ability persists until the volume of functioning liver is so reduced that even the remaining hypermetabolic portions cannot keep up, and doses finally have to be lowered. Thus, drinkers who have not yet completely charred their livers can be given industrial-strength doses of sedatives with almost no calming effect. The same dose given to a nondrinker would calm him down for good in a matter of seconds. I've seen drinkers wide awake after 75 mg of Valium IV given over an hour. If I took the same dose I'd be so sedated that I'd stop breathing and wind up attached to a respirator in the intensive care unit for three weeks.

Mr. Mendez got 100 and another 100 and another 100 over an hour and it still took three people to hold him down, most of whom were sweating and swearing because he'd torn their shirts. After 300 we got nervous that it was all going to kick in suddenly and stop his breathing, forcing us to plug him into a respirator. Though this wasn't a rational fear, we were worried because we knew the same dose might easily kill someone else. Finally, we decided to stop pussyfooting around. The man would either calm down, respirator or no, or fight until his guts wound up all over the walls. We hit him and hit him and hit him, reaching doses of true elephant-stopping dimensions, until the patient settled into relative calmness, babbling quietly with unseen ghosts. He never stopped breathing.

The amazing thing was that Mr. Mendez survived. I remained on the surgical service about two more weeks, during which time he was paid constant attention. There was a member of the housestaff at his bedside virtually twenty-four hours a day. We dumped kilograms of pentobarb and antibiotics into his veins and rinsed out his pancreas with hundreds of liters of sterile saline solution. The sweet smell of pseudomonas eased and his florid jittering and hallucinations disappeared.

I left the surgical service while the patient still had his abdomen open to the breeze. About two months later I decided to stop in and see how he was doing. I walked to the surgical floor and found him in a regular room sitting in bed reading a newspaper. He was shirtless and I noted that the horrible intra-abdominal catastrophe had been reduced to a moderately ugly but well-healed surgical scar extending the length of his belly. On seeing me come in, he put down his paper and smiled.

I said, "How're you doing, Mr. Mendez?"

He responded in accented English, "I'm okay, thanks God, Dr. Intern."

I was surprised that he knew my name. I didn't remember even introducing myself to him. During the period I helped in his care, introducing myself to a blabbering man off in outer space with DTs didn't seem necessary.

I said, "It's good to see you're feeling better."

"Yes, thanks God to you and the other doctors," he replied.

I remembered sticking the IV into his radial artery and sweating and grunting trying to keep him from popping his guts out, a scene that didn't fit my image of well-planned or -conducted medical care, and felt embarrassed.

I said, "Planning on doing any drinking when you get out of here?" and he replied, "No, Doctor, no more drinking for me."

I said, "Glad to hear it. Take care."

He smiled again. "Okay. You take care, too, Doctor." And I walked out of the room. I still sometimes wonder what he's up to today.

The mutilation of millions of livers and pancreases annually by alcoholic Americans is not the only ill consequence of their habit. Another pastime of the big-time boozer is to get really boozed up and drive a car at high velocity until an appropriate object is found to smash into. One of my friends, an orthopedic surgeon, has spent years helping patch up broken drunks and their victims.

He has become a little tired of such less than responsible behavior.

One day, after working in the emergency room, he told me, "After a while you get tired of these guys who come into the ER saying, 'I'm a real fuckin' man now, pal, because you know what I did? I got really fuckin' drunk and went out and totaled my car and myself and a few other people. So now I'm a real fuckin' man.'"

Sometimes drunks are so damn drunk they don't need a drop of anesthesia to be patched up. I've put hundreds of sutures into dozens of drunks without using any local anesthesia at all. The boozer is usually in a fairly good mood when he comes into the ER, full of drunken flamboyancy and covered with blood. Sometimes, especially when repairing a drunk's face, he must be told to stop being so damn gregarious and to shut up or he'll have a crooked smile for the rest of his life. The reply to this is often, "Hey! Jeez, a crooked schmile, that might be kinda intreshting, doc. Yeah, gimme a crooked schmile."

6

Just Say No?

Cigarettes and alcohol are by far the number one killers of Americans, and have probably been so since the discovery of penicillin. A conservative estimate would be that, combined, smoking and booze kill a good 400,000 United States citizens a year; a less conservative estimate would be twice that number. This is interesting, but other than the occasional one-column, page-28 article in *The New York Times,* and a poorly worded "warning" on the side of cigarette packets, this fact gets almost no press. AIDS, in contrast, has reached the top of the disease hit parade after knocking off a measly 30,000 Americans (at the time of this writing) over the last decade. Accepting the worst-case scenario AIDS might kill a million folks in the United States by the turn of the century. In that time smoking and drinking will have slaughtered somewhere between 5 million and 10 million and left twice that number crippled with heart, lung, and liver disease. It's not that I'm upset by the amount of press AIDS has been getting, but rather that I'm perplexed about who decides what it is that we should all get so excited about.

As concern has mounted about AIDS, there has been a resurgence in public awareness of illegal drug abuse. For about ten years, during the period Jimmy Carter so aptly dubbed one of "national malaise," we heard almost noth-

102

ing about junkies. Beginning around 1982, a growing, yet still dim public awareness developed that, yes, drugs were still with us. There was a brief burst of excitement about "angel dust," claimed by some to be a horse tranquilizer and renowned for its ability to endow its frenzied users with the superhuman powers necessary to live out their twisted hallucinations. Angel dust faded when, overnight, "crack" became the instant new star. People marveled at its capacity to render the first-time experimenter into an instant addict. In the last year, prodded by the unavoidable fact that junkies will soon be cluttering the morgues and potter's fields with their emaciated, AIDS-ravaged bodies, the ever fickle public eye has refocused on good old intravenous drug abuse, or, simply, "shooting up." Now we listen to Nancy Reagan, sitting in a house protected by ground-to-air missiles, exhort junkies to "just say no." Gee, things have progressed incredibly, haven't they?

Of course, drugs have been with us all along, and junkies have been dropping like flies whether the public pays attention or not. Sticking oneself with a dirty needle was a dangerous pursuit way before AIDS was invented, although it was, admittedly, a danger limited to the junkie alone. Now that it's been discovered that junkies can spread AIDS as easily with their penises as with their needles, I'm forced to wonder if somewhere in the "just say no" crowd there might be some concern about an accidental encounter with a dangerous penis, as well as concern about humanity in general.

The abuse of illegal drugs comprises another gigantic category in the roster of medical problems encountered on the Cloud Pavilion, at NYG, in the borough of Manhattan, in New York City, and in America, not to mention the rest of the world.

As with virtually all of the other problems encountered in the hospital, approaching the problem of illegal drug abuse from a medical perspective was ass backwards. It

103

did little more than enable society to create junkies without killing them immediately. We ensured that the producers of junk continued to have customers. We treated their patrons, snatched them from the brink of junk-induced death, and booted them back into communities of burnt-out buildings, alienation, and poverty where, surprise, surprise, they elected to shoot up once again.

I'd spent whole nights trying to patch horribly scarred junkies; people who had engaged in truly terrifying self-mutilation for years at a time and come in to the hospital with their fifth and sixth and twentieth episodes of horrendous illness. In the morning I walked out of the hospital and stood waiting for the bus staring at a long ago torched tenement across the street and it was glaringly clear to me that this illness is social pathology and not a medical problem. The liberal attitudes I grew up with became the attitudes that I sincerely believed in, even after I'd been case-hardened by internship, even when I didn't give a shit whether my patients lived or died. I don't care what any of the conservative types say. The catastrophic problem of illegal drug abuse in the United States is the fault and responsibility of society, period.

I fantasized, as I stood waiting for the bus, about a utopian society somewhere between the Garden of Eden and Nazi Germany. A place where the sale of street drugs, the holding up of a grocery store, or the rape of a man or a woman is punishable by a bullet to the nape of the neck on the spot. Where a trillion bucks goes to education instead of "Star Wars." Where farmers are subsidized not to grow tobacco instead of not to grow food. A society that would be kicked off by a gigantic nationwide street party featuring the televised execution of the people, many of whom write the laws and run the law enforcement agencies, who have a hand in the multibillion-dollar American narcotics and organized-crime industry.

That I had these feelings doesn't mean that I didn't hate junkies. Junkies were among the most manipulative, venal, outrightly criminal, and narcissistic of all the patients I ever dealt with. A junkie is destructive of himself and everyone around him and will engage in such destructive behavior over and over and over until he is dead or until he has quit.

I treated a thirty-three-year-old man brought into the emergency room at NYG by the Emergency Medical Service (EMS) for a probable heroin overdose. The EMS saved his life on the street with naloxone, a miracle drug that reverses the effects of opiates. A medicine that "actually works." The EMS found him not breathing on the street, pumped him up with naloxone, and he started to breathe again.

One of the nurses in the ER said he looked familiar and I checked to see if he had an old chart at the hospital. I discovered he'd been discharged the week before after spending a few months in the hospital recovering from his previous overdose. The prior hospital course was characterized by his body closing shop almost completely for about three weeks. A breathing machine did his breathing for him, a kidney dialysis machine made his pee-pee for him, antibiotics attacked the bacteria that set up housekeeping all over his body, and drugs maintained his blood pressure at seminormal levels while he slowly recovered.

At first I had trouble believing the patient had chosen to celebrate life by going out and overdosing again. Then, thinking back on the hundreds of times I'd seen such behavior in the past, I realized that I wasn't really so surprised after all.

The man had an ultranew haircut that gave his head the appearance of a layered mushroom. His name was Hispanic but he kept yelling, *"Eh, paisan, capice?"* which is

Italian, and drooling on the floor. Because naloxone had so effectively ended his high, it was clear that he'd been doing that most popular of opiates, heroin. Nonetheless, he continued to behave in a bizarre manner, drifting off to sleep and occasionally waking to slander a passing nurse. I figured he might have been abusing other chemicals in addition to heroin, mixing his pleasures as it were, and that this might account for his still-strange behavior. Who knew what other poisons he might have shot up, eaten, whatever.

The effect of naloxone was only to reverse the physiologic effects of opiates. There was a pharmacopoeia of other substances he might have done, and I was obligated to do my best to completely purge his system. I decided to attack the gastrointestinal port of entry first. His belly might prove a treasure trove of pills: Valiums, Libriums, barbiturates, ups, downs, hallucinogens.

I convinced him to drink 30 cc of ipecac, another in the fantastic class of drugs that actually work; in this case to cause spectacular vomiting.

A quick search of this prize, however, revealed no pill fragments or capsules, so I would now work on the assumption that chemicals unknown were already adrift in his probably AIDS-infected bloodstream. In the name of good medical care, I would next ask the patient to drink a big glassful of charcoal slurry. Charcoal slurry is exactly that, ground up charcoal suspended in water. It looks disgusting but doesn't taste like anything at all. It helps pill overdosers by providing an absolutely tremendous surface area for sucking up whatever might be left in their intestines. It can even suck bad stuff out of the blood right through the intestine walls. Once it has sucked up everything in sight, it holds the chemicals in a miserly grip until the whole mess passes out of the other end of the patient.

The process of passing the mess out the other end of

the patient is hastened with a bottle of magnesium citrate, which causes a tremendous case of the shits. All of the charcoal and any remaining pills are blown clean out of the patient.

Mag citrate is used before special X-ray tests of the intestines where it is undesirable for shit to show up on the films, and in people who have eaten something bad that has to be gotten out of their system as fast as possible. Causing the shits is an efficacious way of accomplishing both ends. Vomiting alone isn't good enough to clear the system because given time the stuff gets squeezed down past the stomach in the normal process of digestion, and barfing will no longer expel it.

Despite my well-intentioned plans, the patient now decided to stop cooperating, though "cooperation" did not best describe his earlier behavior, either. Mostly he'd slobbered, yelled obscenities, and shrieked, *"Eh, paisan, capice?"* He was behaving typically, making a nuisance of himself, seemingly unaware of the damage his habit was doing himself, and unwilling to see his own role in his predicament. It was a form of behavior a shrink would call a character disorder, in which an individual is unwilling or unable to assume responsibility for his own actions, and manipulates others to assume that responsibility. This patient was too stupid for conscious manipulation but had succeeded to engage the attention of doctors, nurses, the EMS, the police, his family, and probably a number of others, as well as to spend a good six figures of public money in his care.

I'd cajoled him into taking the ipecac by saying, "Listen, pal, I'm only interested in helping you here, and if you don't want to be helped why don't you just drink this stuff so that I can say I've done my job properly, and stop giving me such a pain in the ass?"

Junkies often respond favorably to blunt honesty and he'd decided, after a few more bouts of obscenity and drooling, to drink the ipecac. I don't think he suspected the sly doctor of causing the sudden wave of nausea and vomiting that overcame him. Nonetheless, he subsequently refused to behave. Lying diagonally across the stretcher, his legs hanging off one side and his head off the other, drool dripping into his mushroom haircut, he elected only to yell, "*Eh! Paisan! Capice?* Fucking asshole! *Capice?*"

I sat down to consider my next move. The options were pretty straightforward: I'd either force treatment on the patient, or let the issue pass. Because he had intentionally overdosed I didn't have to take no for an answer. There were a number of solid legal arguments backing forced treatment, arguments I'll get into in more detail when I discuss the patient who has attempted suicide. I could simply ask the ER cops to hold the patient down, and force a plastic tube through his nose, down his throat, and into his belly. I'd then pour the charcoal and magnesium citrate into him regardless of his degree of cooperation. It would be a nice, emphatic way to vent the anger and frustration I was feeling about his behavior. Unfortunately, such scenes can get ugly, with the patient flailing all over the stretcher knocking things off of tables, trying to bite people, and spraying blood and snot all over the place.

When the patient first came in I'd sent a sample of his blood for a toxicology screen, a few random stabs in the dark that might identify what he had taken. The results revealed that his blood was free of alcohol, barbiturates, aspirin, and Tylenol; the first two very common drugs of abuse, the latter two lethal favorites among the suicide crowd. In all likelihood I'd never find out what else he'd used, cocaine, PCP, whatever. I could spend a few hundred dollars of public money running esoteric assays on his blood for these substances, but because they lacked long-term sequelae, it didn't make any difference if they were identified. That the patient was gradually becoming more and more alert, rather than more and more sleepy, was also encouraging. Whatever it was, it wasn't having a deepening effect on him.

In addition, the patient had no evidence of trauma to his head. Head trauma is a common cause of deepening lethargy in the sleepy patient, and obligates the doctor to order a CAT scan to search for bleeding inside the skull. New York's taxpayers would be saved that expense (on the order of $300-$500) as well.

I finally decided to let the whole thing pass. I just wasn't in the mood for more ugliness. I left the ER a few hours later with a vague, uneasy sense that the patient would box two or three days down the line because I'd failed to realize what esoteric poison he'd taken and take the steps necessary to get it out of him. About a month and a half later he overdosed again, fell and cut his head, and came in to get stitches. I recognized him while the surgeon was sewing him up, and thought, "How do you like that, he didn't die after all." Too bad, really.

When treating people like this, my reaction was to get angry. Others felt the same. While the patient was draped over the stretcher drooling into his hair and yelling obscenities, one of the nurses asked if she could go over and strangle him. I said, "Fine by me!"

I got particularly angry when the patient had just started shooting up. It was one thing to use needles when the worst that could happen was addiction, a life of misery, a number of horrible (though usually curable) medical complications, and a violent drug-related death. AIDS has changed things completely. In the Bronx, for example, the AIDS virus (known on the street as "the virus") has infected somewhere between 50 and 90 percent of junkies, the majority of whom share needles. The chance of the beginning junkie getting infected is catastrophically high.

It's like playing Russian roulette with five bullets. The odds are the hammer ain't going to land on the empty barrel.

A young girl no more than eighteen years old came in to the ER one day, sobbing and streaming tears, and explained that in the last three weeks she'd gone from experimenting with heroin to getting hooked. "Please, oh, please, Doctor," she begged, "help me get off and take away the withdrawal pain." I told her that if she were my sister I'd solve the problem by beating her into next week and sitting on her for twenty-four hours while she yawned and fidgeted herself into a state of drug freedom. Instead, I gave her a small dose of methadone, enough to take the edge off withdrawal, and referred her to a rehab program. I wonder how she did.

Another in an endless procession of junkies was a young overdoser, maybe eighteen years old, with five or ten fresh needle marks and no old scars. He arrived in the ER unconscious and, despite being stuck with a needle and injected with naloxone, failed to wake up. Since naloxone only works on opiates, this was conclusive evidence that he'd been mixing his pleasures (polydrug abuse). Something else was making him sleepy and, unlike the case of his mushroom-topped cohort (who did wake up with naloxone), purging his gastrointestinal system, pouring in charcoal, and giving him a ferocious case of diarrhea with mag citrate was absolutely indicated. Failing to do everything possible to remove whatever was causing his lethargy would amount to medical negligence.

Despite my fondness for ipecac, the patient's drowsy condition forbade its use. Giving a sleeping patient ipecac risks vomiting and aspiration. Forcing a sleeping person to throw up and then choke on his vomit is a prime example of a medical screwup (an "iatrogenic" illness, one resulting from a doctor's actions). Though junkies made me feel frustrated and angry, I had no intention of working out my anger by getting vomit into this kid's lungs. The pneumonia that results can be really horrible.

Thorny as it is, the problem of the drowsy patient in need of a good stomach pumping and intestinal steam cleaning has a nifty solution. It is called gastric lavage. First, the patient is "intubated"; a tube (called an endotracheal, or ET, tube) is stuck into his mouth and wedged into his windpipe. Usually this is done for respiratory failure, and the tube is attached to a machine that breathes for the patient. In gastric lavage, it serves a different purpose: the creation of a protected airway. The only way in or out of the patient's lungs is through the tube.

Once intubated, the patient is assaulted with an Ewald tube. This tube is about the diameter of a garden hose, easily wide enough to accommodate whatever is in the patient's gizzards, even intact pills. It is reamed down the patient's throat and into his belly, and a suction machine is attached to vacuum out the gastric contents. Then, after the stomach is thoroughly drained, washed, rinsed, and spin-dried, the charcoal slurry and magnesium citrate are poured in and the Ewald tube removed. The patient spends a minute or two gagging, spitting, and vomiting (the garden hose placement and removal procedure being very unpleasant to all but the deeply comatose) and, after he calms down and there is no further risk of vomiting and aspiration, the endotracheal tube is removed. *Voilá!* The well-managed overdose patient.

Naturally, this management plan is not without its difficulties, one of which is its dependence on intubation. Tubing is an exceedingly scary and uncomfortable procedure for all but the genuinely unconscious or dead, and patients who aren't completely out rarely allow it without a fight. In fact, the easiest patient to tube is a dead one. At cardiac arrests, patients are immediately intubated and administered oxygen with a manually compressed balloon. Not only is this the best way to deliver oxygen to a dead

111

person, but it saves the staff the necessity of doing mouth to mouth on someone who may have died of some particularly vicious form of pneumonia.

The young man in question fit into the category of not quite comatose. I figured he might put up a bit of a ruckus when I tried to tube him, and called the anesthesiologist ("gas man") to come down to the ER in case I needed help. Anesthesiologists are the last word in intubation. Together, we spent about a half hour trying to get the tube in, while the patient gagged and squirmed mightily. Several times he put on a terrific show of turning purple and choking as though he were about to give up on breathing altogether. This, admittedly, would have made the task much easier. Finally, it became clear that my plan was doomed to failure. The only possible solution was to sedate the patient to stop his struggling, but this seemed a bit ridiculous when drug-induced lethargy was the problem to start with.

The whole scene was so traumatic that the poor fellow eventually woke up a bit. I decided that he'd have to wake up some more and either tell me what drugs he'd done, or drink the ipecac and commence throwing up, or both.

I sat him up and yelled into his face, "What did you take?!"

He opened his eyes halfway. "Nothing." He slumped back down on the stretcher.

Suddenly, I became furious. An idiot kid who'd just started shooting up in total disregard to both himself and his family, who'd probably come within minutes of losing his life, and who was now slobbering all over his shirt, was telling the doctor he had done "nothing." I sat him up again and, holding him by the collar with one hand, slapped him hard across the face.

"Wake up!" I yelled. "What did you take?!"

He didn't answer so I smacked him again, much harder, making him flinch. I was about to yell again when

112

I realized that I was shaking. The nurse who'd been assisting with the patient looked up at me. Her eyes said she knew what I was feeling, and that she was feeling it too, but that it was time to stop. I released his collar, my hand still raised in the air, let him slump back down on the stretcher, and went to gather my things and go home, as my shift had ended. I never found out what happened to him after I left.

Despite the frustration inherent in dealing with junkies, I found it interesting to ask about details of their lives. I didn't know, before I started dealing with junkies, how all-consuming junk could be, that it could completely take over an addict's life. I was surprised again and again, as I asked more questions, by the extraordinary things they did to support their habits. Miss Davis had had sex with thousands of strangers. Others admitted to mugging, burglary, even murder, all for the same reason, all in the name of junk.

One of the interesting things about being a doctor was the kinds of details people offered about their lives. Were I to walk up to someone on the subway wearing a pair of shorts and a T-shirt and ask, "How many people would you say you've had sex with in your life, rounding off to the nearest ten?" I'd have a good chance of getting punched in the mouth. But, when I was in the hospital wearing my doctor costume, I'd get an honest reply to this question. I often asked more than was called for because the things people said were so interesting. Professional doctor critics will yell and scream that this is not ethical, but I don't care. It was fascinating and I never betrayed anyone's confidence.

I might ask a junkie, "So, do you work?"

Most didn't.

Then I'd ask, "How do you get along?"

They'd reply, "Oh, you know, I get around."

I'd say, "No really, I don't know, what does 'getting around' mean?"

Usually it meant burglary or the like. After listening to detailed descriptions of sundry break-ins and muggings I'd say, "Well, listen, if you ever find yourself in an apartment and you see something with my name on it, how about you return the favor for my caring for you here in the hospital by just leaving, okay?" They'd smile and nod their heads. I guess it didn't work, because while I lived in New York City my apartment was broken into three times.

I was particularly intrigued by people's tattoos. In the middle of an interview I'd notice a name tattooed on a guy's arm and ask, "Who's that?"

The answer might be, "Oh, that's this girl I know."

I'd continue asking medical questions and, after a while, ask, "So, you still know her or what?"

The patient might answer, "No, we broke up a few years ago, but we lived together for a while."

I'd say, "Yeah? What happened?" and the patient would spend ten minutes telling me about this past love and why it didn't work out.

I asked one guy about a tattoo and was told he got it after killing someone. I suppose it was like the symbols World War II air aces painted on their airplanes whenever they shot down one of the enemy. I asked the patient if he'd been arrested for this crime and he matter-of-factly informed me that he had, and spent ten years in jail. I decided not to ask about the rest of his tattoos.

Another man who came into the ER had the names of his wife and two daughters inscribed on his arm. He returned a few months later when one of his daughters accidentally cut herself. He walked the little girl into the exam room and she burst into tears.

I pointed at the names on her daddy's arm. "This one's

114

your mommy and this is your sister, right?"

Her eyes lit up in amazement and she stopped crying.

I said, "See? Doctors know lots of things!" and winked at her father. He didn't remember me from his prior visit and asked how I knew the meaning of the names on his arm.

I told him I had an eye for tattoos.

Drug abuse has long been an impetus for bizarre behavior. Because of its association with AIDS, intravenous drug abuse, or IVDA, has become the current darling of the popular press. This doesn't mean, of course, that the smoking, eating, and snorting of drugs, and all the destructive sequelae of these behaviors, no longer exist. It's just that other topics are currently more in vogue.

"Intravenous drug abuse," incidentally, is the correct and appropriate medical phrase for this habit, and not "intravenous drug use," a term now popular among the defenders of junkies. When a junkie sticks himself with a needle and shoots in dope, he is engaging in abuse, plain and simple. Further, as derogatory as it is, I see little wrong with the word "junkie." Those who insist on the phrases "intravenous drug use" and "user" claim that the other terms, "abuse" and "junkie," denigrate people who are victims. As far as I'm concerned there is no reason to dance around the edge of the issue. There is no respect to be afforded this behavior, and no reason to use neutral terms in referring to those who engage in it. That a junkie is a victim, that there are reasons external to the junkie himself that have driven him to junk, that he is in desperate need of help, and inhabits the body of a normal, productive human being doesn't mean he isn't a junkie. It's a word that bluntly and clearly identifies his habit as the horrible and self-destructive action that it is. We don't call murderers "perpetrators of lethal violence,"

115

or rapists "sexual assaulters," despite a widely held view that many such people are in desperate need of help. Why insist on a neutral phrase for people who murder and rape their own bodies?

One of the most famous nonintravenous drugs for generating stories about bizarre behavior was phencyclidine: "angel dust," or "PCP." Although little is heard anymore about angel dust, it was well known for its ability to both addle and confer superhuman powers upon its abusers, or so the stories went. Tales of "some guy who was dusted" going berserk and beating up six cops before fifteen more managed to subdue him abounded. In my work at NYG, I witnessed some exceedingly strange dust-induced behavior, including one patient who'd done the most bizarre thing to himself I'd ever seen or heard of in my life.

This man smoked dust one day and surprised his friends by politely excusing himself to the bathroom, bringing along his two Doberman pinschers. In the bathroom he opened the medicine cabinet, removed a straight-edge razor, cut off his own facial features one by one, and fed them to his dogs. He emerged from the bathroom with no ears, nose, eyelids, lips, or cheeks, and two happy-looking dogs.

His friends, now fairly distraught, brought him to the NYG emergency room, where the plastic and head and neck surgeons pissed in their pants with excitement. They took him straight to the operating room. Jokes emerged immediately. The man lost face, the surgeons tried to save face, etc., etc.

In order to create a new face for this unfortunate patient, the surgeons did a "pectoral flap," a fascinating procedure in which the pectoral (chest) muscle is removed and reimplanted at another site on a patient's body. The surgeons don't remove the muscle completely, but leave intact its main artery and vein. The muscle is then "flapped" to the spot where it's needed, presumably a hole

116

that is too deep to be filled by mere skin grafting, and sewn in place. Eventually, it grows a new blood supply at the transplant site and the surgeons remove the original artery and vein. The man with no face had two pectoral flaps done, one from each side of his chest to each side of his face. Once the muscles were well established in their new locations the surgeons took him back to the OR about two hundred times to cut and shape and revise the graft to create a new face for him.

I know the story of the man with no face is true because I saw him walking down the hall a few weeks after he was admitted. He was wearing a surgical hood turned back in the front, with two holes cut out for his eyes, like the "elephant man."

I whispered to a coresident, "Who's that?"

He looked at me with wide eyes. "That's the man with no face!"

It was the most bizarre story I'd ever heard.

Another hideous story about angel dust describes the unfortunate young woman who was brought into the NYG emergency room with massive vaginal bleeding. The patient was bleeding so fiercely that the gynecologists carted her off immediately to the operating room. After cleaning up all the blood in her crotch, they found a loop of intestine hanging from her vagina. The loop of gut extended right up through a torn cervix into the uterus, through a hole in the uterine wall, and up into the abdominal cavity. The surgeons cut a hole in the woman's abdomen and, reaching down from above the uterus, tugged the loop of intestine back into its proper place. Then they patched the injuries in the uterus and cervix and closed her belly.

After the woman awoke from surgery she was asked what happened. She and her boyfriend were smoking angel dust and messing around, she explained, and she remembered his fondling of her genitalia suddenly becoming excruciatingly painful, and looking down to see all this blood. The surgeons surmised that the boyfriend forced his hand up into her vagina, through the cervix, into the uterus, and through the uterine wall, where he grabbed a loop of intestine and pulled it back down and out before letting go. The patient had literally had her guts ripped out. The phrase the surgeons used was "manually eviscerated."

Perhaps the story of the man with no face wasn't the strangest I ever heard after all.

One of the last reasons for substance abuse is the intention to cause harm. Suicide successes, attempts, and so-called gestures are extremely popular, and to ingest a substance believed to be toxic is perhaps the most popular method. I've seen very few successful, and many unsuccessful suicides. This probably reflects the fact that people who don't really intend to die ensure they will wind up in the hospital for treatment, while those who wish to die merely take the pills and go to sleep, or pull the trigger, or jump off the bridge, and don't tell anybody about it.

The people who drive the morgue trucks have all the good stories about successful suicide attempts. There is, in fact, an actual museum of death in New York City, down at the Office of the Chief Medical Examiner. It features the pertinent body parts, preserved forever in jars of formalin, of people who died in any number of gruesomely fascinating ways.

There is, for example, the young fellow who successfully urinated on the third rail in the subway when dared to do so by his friends. He was electrocuted immediately, and his shriveled penis sits in a jar in the museum of death, an explicit, graphic reminder of his youthful indiscretion. Included in the penis section is the member belonging to the poor fellow who was completely disfigured

118

in an automobile accident, and positively identified when his tearful wife recognized his penis.

No tale of the Office of the Chief Medical Examiner is complete without the story of the unfortunate rookie cop who shot and killed a crook on his first day on the force. After the smoke of the shoot-out cleared and the body was removed, the cop was taken down to the ME's office to positively identify the man as the one he killed. He was received by the ME's PR man, a fellow who, unfortunately, took to hunching his back, rubbing his hands, and speaking in tones reminiscent of Peter Lorre whenever he brought a visitor down to the morgue. He led the nervous officer downstairs and, rubbing his hands amidst the cadavers lying on their classic oversized file drawers, excused himself to run off and collect the ME, who was in the adjoining autopsy room. While electric buzz saws ground and stuttered in the near distance, busy at their unpleasant tasks, the cop stood nervously shifting and glancing about, completely alone in the morgue room.

No one, of course, had informed the officer of the fact that the freshly dead will, on occasion, move. Although such movement is usually limited to reflex twitches, perhaps the bending of a finger, or even the flexing of an elbow, it is not unheard of for a body to make a significant movement, like sitting up.

As the cop stood waiting and fidgeting, a nearby body had the audacity to do just that. It sat up. The cadaver's motion forced its abdominal viscera up against its diaphragm, compressing the lung cavity and causing it to emit an audible "Uhhh . . ." The cop whipped around to find himself face to face with a dead man. Sitting in a slumped position, the corpse regarded him with dull, dead, glazed eyes.

Now, let's remember that the cop had had a remarkably bad first day on the job, and therefore that he was considerably on edge. He drew his revolver, already used once in the day, assumed a crouched shooting position, and emptied all six chambers into the corpse. "BLAM! BLAM! BLAM! BLAM! BLAM! BLAM!"

The sound of busy buzz saws halted immediately, and a half-dozen people clad in bloody aprons rushed from the autopsy room into the morgue. The cop, still in a crouched position, stared at the corpse wild-eyed, his smoking gun shaking visibly but aimed squarely at its chest. The body remained in a sitting position, still regarding the officer dully, with six neat, unbleeding bullet holes in its chest and abdomen. The autopsy room staff broke into hysterical laughter.

I never found out if the cop remained on the force.

One of the surest ways to die is to take a fistful of Tylenol and not seek medical care. About twenty-four to thirty-six hours later a drawn-out, painful, and irreversible death is guaranteed from massive liver failure. One of the few suicide successes I saw resulted from a Tylenol overdose. Tylenol (generic name, "acetaminophen") is a double-edged sword being not only deadly but also a favorite among adolescents wishing to make a "suicide gesture." A kid may take a handful and not let on until too late, thinking the stuff is harmless. I place the term "suicide gesture" in quotation because any mental health professional (shrink) will note in very grave tones that talk of suicide in a teenager is serious business.

Almost all the suicide attempts I've seen were in young women between the ages of fifteen and thirty-five who were entangled in complex home lives. The stories ranged from the insipid and trivial, as with fifteen-year-olds distraught over estranged boyfriends, to horrific, though common, tales of rape and other physical (and emotional) violence committed against women of all ages.

For those of us with jaded hearts, those whose souls had

been cracked by internship, many of the things people did to themselves in the name of suicide seemed amusing, even in the most horrible of circumstances. Unquestionably, this reaction was partly the result of some sort of psychologic defense mechanism, designed to protect us from the anguish we dealt with on a daily basis. Nonetheless, it is also true that much of what we saw really was amusing.

One day, I treated a young woman in the NYC ER who had washed down a handful of Tylenol with a few swigs of Clorox. The patient, who was very upset, cried copiously and, with each wail, wafted the scent of Clorox into my face. I remember the odd, distinct sensation that her breath smelled like a freshly scrubbed toilet. I was impressed by the woman's emotional resolve, one so forceful that she actually chugged a bottle of laundry bleach.

The combination she'd chosen, Clorox and Tylenol, created a nifty paradox in management. The problem was whether to leave the Tylenol in her belly and chance liver failure, or risk burns to the esophagus (Clorox being caustic) were she made to vomit. Eventually, I decided to use sedation, intubation, and an Ewald tube to clean her out, a plan which obviated both possibilities. Being still distraught, the patient refused to comply until I told her that, by intending to kill herself, she had lost a number of her civil rights. She would cooperate or I'd ask five or six big, burly policemen to hold her down while I did my dirty work regardless of her wishes.

Those who think this unfair might first consider the options in this situation. The alternative was allowing a twenty-five-year-old woman to die. They may also consider the answer to the question, inevitably posed by the attorney for the patient's family, "Why exactly, Doctor, did the patient die while under your care?"

I had a friend who worked for the NYC EMS for several years before he went to medical school. He was loaded with weird and true stories about the things he saw on the streets of New York. His favorite was about a guy who committed suicide by jumping out a window. I heard him tell the story a few times.

A young man was involved in a discussion with his sweetheart about the depth of his love for her. She claimed he didn't love her sufficiently, and he that his love was without bound, that he would do anything she asked. His lover laughed and said this could not possibly be true. For example, he would not throw himself out of the window on her command, would he? All she need do, he responded, was tell him to do so. She did, and so did he. My friend and his partner arrived to find the young man and his brains lying at two different spots on the sidewalk. My friend couldn't help laughing in an apologetic, perplexed way every time he told this story.

The story didn't end with his wiping the patient and his brains off the sidewalk. He and his partner brought the body (and the brains) to the hospital to be declared dead. They carted him into the emergency room of some city hospital and fetched an intern. They unwrapped the body and the intern, apparently quite new, began to listen with a stethoscope for a heartbeat. My friend decided to let him do his thing. He didn't point out that a physically brainless patient is very unlikely to have a heartbeat.

But, there's more. The intern finally decided the patient had boxed. Headed for Cloud 9. My buddy carted the patient down to the hospital morgue, where a pathologist sat smoking a cigarette and reading a magazine. When the body arrived his eyes lit up.

He said, "Whatcha got here?" and listened to the man's unfortunate story, his eyes getting ever brighter.

On its completion he exclaimed, "You mean this guy and his brains are in two separate pieces?! Lemme see!"

The body was again unwrapped and the pathologist

said, "Wait a minute!" and disappeared. He returned a minute later with a camera and flash unit and took several frenzied shots of the body with a few close-ups of the brains.

My pal, a bit flabbergasted, said, "What are you doing?"

The pathologist replied, "It's for my collection. Come in next week and I'll show it to you!"

As it turned out, my friend happened to be quite unintentionally back in the same hospital exactly one week later and bumped into the pathologist in the hallway.

The doc said, "Hey! I've been looking forward to seeing you! Come on downstairs and I'll show you my album." Before my friend could reply, he grabbed him by the sleeve and led him back down to the morgue where he showed him a photo album full of color photos of mutilated corpses. My friend described it as a collection worthy of the museum of death itself.

7

Successes

Mrs. Sweet was an old lady who loved me. I loved her, too, although I don't remember at all how this love affair began. All I remember is that she was my patient at the clinic where I worked a few afternoons a week, she never missed an appointment, and it was always wonderful to see her.

Mrs. Sweet's primary medical problem was her history of recurrent benign brain tumors. She'd had three tumors over the course of ten or fifteen years, and three operations to have them removed. She also had diabetes, or maybe it was hypertension, and was referred to my clinic for these nonneurologic problems. Neurosurgeons are very skilled, but never stray from the nervous system.

It seems fairly obvious that anyone who has his skull opened up three times is going to be left with permanent damage, no matter how skilled his surgeon. Mrs. Sweet had done fine after her first two operations, but developed some pretty severe problems after the third. Amazingly, however, I'm not suggesting that her surgeon was at fault. As I said, damage is bound to happen after so many operations, and the surgeon had clearly saved her life not once, but three times.

The damage, which involved the visual system, was very obvious. She was permanently walleyed and totally blind on the left, and had lost most of her peripheral vision on the right. In sum, her eyesight was limited to a small patch of sight in the center of her line of vision in the right eye. These deficits had probably resulted from injuries to the nerves controlling vision and the movement of the eyes. These nerves are a part of the system of twelve cranial nerves, which control not only vision, but all the things that heads and faces do: movement of the tongue, taste, facial expressions, eyeball movement, hearing, smell, and many other functions. (A famous medical student dirty joke concerns the cranial nerves. It goes, "What do the chorda tympani branch of the seventh cranial nerve and the clitoris have in common?" The answer is, "They both provide taste to the anterior two thirds of the tongue," which I think I'll leave unexplained.)

That Mrs. Sweet had serious visual difficulties is not to say that she wasn't terrific or that I didn't love her. All it meant was that she needed a little more time than most to negotiate certain tasks, and that every once in a while she bumped into something that she hadn't seen because it was out of her line of sight. I refilled her medicines regularly, whether they were for diabetes or high blood pressure, and she took them religiously.

Naturally, I was very concerned when Mrs. Sweet showed up one day without an appointment to tell me that she had started to suffer from roaring headaches.

Headaches, it almost goes without saying, are a primary symptom of brain tumors. A tension headache, which results from tensing the muscles of the face or sides of the head, causes widespread, or "generalized," dull or throbbing pain. But, if a patient says, "Jeez, Doc, this pain feels like a goddam knife sticking in right behind my left eyeball," then a tumor is a possibility. Tumors can be located just about anywhere, and often cause asymmetric sharp pain, rather than generalized dull pain. It is also important to ask whether the patient has ever had that

125

kind of headache before. If they say, "Yeah, but it hasn't been this bad since I went through my divorce two years ago," then a tumor is less likely.

Mrs. Sweet tended to get headaches and seizures every time she had a brain tumor, poor lady, and that was why I was so concerned when she came in complaining about a headache. I didn't go through all the tumor versus non-tumor headache questions though, because she knew the differences very well and because she'd have to see the surgeon no matter what the answers.

"Doctor," she said, "I'm worried. I'm just so worried. I've been having those headaches again." Even though she had rushed in to see me without an appointment, she still wore her Sunday best, which she always did when she came to the clinic. She even wore a big ornate hat with that mesh veil that older women seem to like so much, and a big ribbon.

I came right to the point. "Do they feel like the headaches you had before the tumors?"

She nodded her head. "Oh, dear, oh yes they do, Doctor, I'm so worried."

I said, "Now you know that you're one of my favorite patients, but you also know that I'm not an expert at this, and you must immediately go see Dr. Neuron, your neurologist, or Dr. Neurosurgeon, your neurosurgeon. They're the experts in this. I'll call and get you an appointment immediately."

I had a habit of calling to make appointments for my patients when they needed to see consultants. This took up a tremendous amount of time, but a whole lot less than it took them to do it themselves, and it also cut about two months off the waiting period. That was one of the things that being a doc was great for; it really helped cut down on time spent fighting on the phone with secretaries. Even when I took care of personal business on the phone, I'd get to whoever I was calling fifty times faster when I said, "This is Dr. Intern calling," rather than simply giving my name. Sometimes the person who answered the phone would say, "I'm sorry, but Mr. So-and-so isn't in. May I take a message?" I'd say, "Yeah, uh, just tell him Dr. Intern called and to please call back as soon as possible." Then there'd be a pause followed by, "Oh, he just stepped in, hold on a second and I'll put you through."

Mrs. Sweet looked very distressed. "Oh, Doctor, now, they just never have the time to see me. Can't you take care of this for me instead of making me see that other doctor?"

I said, "You know I can't do that, so let me call Dr. Neuron right now and get you an appointment." I didn't let her argue with me, and picked up the phone to call the neurologist.

It took only four calls to get the correct number, and then five minutes on hold to get through to Dr. Neuron.

I finally hung up. "Okay, Mrs. Sweet, here's what you have to do. Dr. Neuron is arranging for you to get a CAT scan first thing in the morning. Then you're going to his office in the afternoon to find out the results."

She looked really forlorn. "Oh, Doctor, can't I get the results from you?"

I said, "It's much better to get the results from Dr. Neuron, because he's the expert. I wouldn't want to make a mistake looking at your CAT scan. That would make me feel terrible. Please go and see Dr. Neuron tomorrow."

Mrs. Sweet examined a three-foot patch of the floor with her one functioning eye. "Well, I guess I have to do whatever is necessary."

Mrs. Sweet left after I gave her a prescription for some painkillers for her headache and then didn't keep her doctor's appointment the following day. Instead she called me at the clinic.

"I'm so sorry," she said. "But I just couldn't go in to see

127

that other doctor. Did you look at my X ray?"

I thought for a second about getting mad at her, but decided against it. "No I didn't. I thought you'd be with Dr. Neuron and he'd tell you. What happened?"

"Well, oh dear, couldn't you just go in and look at it for me?" Her forlorn look radiated over the phone.

I said, "Okay. I'll call you later this evening," and went to the radiology suite at MH to find Mrs. Sweet's CAT scan after I finished at the clinic.

Most of the radiology residents had fled into radiology after being horror-stricken by the third year of medical school. The third year is pretty hairy, and scares off a fair chunk of each class from not only patient care, but medicine as a whole. Unfortunately, the investment of time and energy is too great to simply quit altogether and start driving a cab, so some students flee into the no-patient-contact specialties. These include radiology ("rads"), nuclear medicine ("unclear medicine" or "nukes"), and pathology ("path"). Some people decide they still sort of like the idea of dealing with patients, but don't want to get too intense or bloody and go into dermatology ("derm") or rehabilitation medicine ("rehab"). Some figure they still like blood but also want to get home by five, and go into "invasive radiology," where they get to stick catheters deep into people's bodies, release dyes, and take all sorts of neat X rays of their brains and spleens and kidneys.

The radiology department at MH was far away from any of the clinical floors, and was filled with little tiny dark cubicles. Each cubicle had one wall covered with a special light cabinet gizmo that held around two hundred X rays. The radiologists would sit in front and read the X rays and dictate the reports into tape recorders. Whenever you went down to the radiology suite to get an X ray read you had to stick your head into one of the little cubicles and interrupt whoever was inside reading films. The old-timers, guys who'd been reading films for fifty years, were usually pretty nice about this, and even took a little interest in the case. The young guys tended to be a bit strange about it. They'd look at you like you were from Mars because of all the piss and vomit on your white pants, and you could just about hear them thinking, "But for the grace of God, there goes me." Since they didn't have to deal with piss and vomit they were fairly snappy dressers, and looked like miniattendings. They also behaved like it was a major sacrifice to read a film for you. If you were on call and needed an emergency study done in the middle of the night, whichever radiology resident was on would shit himself complaining about it.

I went to the CAT scan part of the radiology suite and found the neuroradiologists reading the head scans. The neuroradiologists had very big opinions of themselves because they read such fancy X rays, and if you came into their little cubicle with blood and shit on your white pants they wouldn't even look at you. I hadn't wanted to go down there at all, except for the fact that I'd told Mrs. Sweet I would. I didn't want to get sneered at by the neurorad people, even though I'd been in clinic and didn't have any shit or blood on my pants. I'd called Dr. Neuron, but he hadn't seen the scan, so I was obligated to find it and get it read myself. When I found the films I stuck them up on one of the light boxes. A group of docs sat nearby reading a bunch of scans and electing not to recognize my presence at all, so I decided to read them on my own. There was relatively little risk in doing this because Dr. Neuron would see them sooner or later, and if there was a problem he'd let me know.

I looked at Mrs. Sweet's brain for fifteen minutes and saw no problems that might be indicative of a recurrent tumor. I put her films back in the jacket and went home.

I called her and said, "Listen, Mrs. Sweet, you know I'm not an expert at this, but I looked at your CAT scan and didn't see a new tumor. I want you to call Dr. Neuron tomorrow and find out what the experts said. Then I want you to come and see me next week so we can see how your headache is doing."

She said, "Oh, Doctor, I feel so much better. I'll be there next week."

She came in the next week in a fresh set of her Sunday best and a particularly frilly hat, looking terrific.

I said, "How are your headaches?"

She replied, "They went away as soon as you told me about the X ray. I feel fine." She told me she felt so good that she never even bothered to call the neurologist. The neurologist never called me, either, so I figured my reading had been accurate.

Mrs. Sweet's blood pressure (or maybe it was her diabetes) was also under perfect control, and she didn't get any more headaches for the rest of my residency. When I finished my training and left the clinic for good she came in for a last appointment. She cried when she said good-bye, and, occasionally, I still wonder how she's doing and if she ever got headaches again. I hope not.

Mr. Johnson was eighty years old and had a blood pressure of 240/150 when he came to see me on his first clinic visit. He'd been living way the hell up in northern Manhattan near the Cloisters just about forever and had been married to his wife even longer. He was a big, sturdy, robust guy, and still worked a part-time job as a messenger at some big downtown firm. The money he earned supplemented his social security and a small pension so that he and his wife had just enough to make ends meet.

Mr. Johnson received no health insurance through his job (I'm not sure of the reason for this, perhaps it was because he was part time, or maybe he worked off the books) and depended solely on Medicare, the federal health insurance program for people over age sixty-five, for his health care needs. Medicare would pay for office visits and hospitalizations (less a deductible and 20 percent of overall charges), but not the cost of outpatient medications. Mr. Johnson earned *too much* money to qualify for Medicaid (the federal health insurance program for the poor) and did not have private insurance, the only other sources of coverage for prescription meds. The cost of medicines can eat up a tremendous chunk of an elderly person's income, and Mr. Johnson simply didn't have the money. At the age of eighty, and still working, he was a member of a class known as the working poor, people who make too much money to qualify for federal assistance, but not enough to afford "luxuries" like decent health insurance. I might add that conservatives who jump up and down screaming that Medicare *is* federal assistance should remember that people like Mr. Johnson have been paying for it in taxes for decades.

The clinic where I worked was unique in having a program that helped "working poor" people pay for their health care needs. There was a sliding scale of charges that ranged from 0 percent (i.e., no charge) to full payment. We also split the cost of many of our patients' medications with them, sometimes paying most or all of the cost. The reason we were able to do this was because we had a bunch of grant money that was designed to help provide health care for poor people. We were not in the medicine-for-profit biz.

Mr. Johnson heard about us by word of mouth, especially our med program, and dragged his ass up on the subway from his messenger job downtown for a visit, knowing he would probably need prescription drugs.

He was right. A blood pressure of 240/150 will raise the hackles on just about any doc, even me. A BP that high is a hairbreadth away from a major stroke. I figured a major stroke was not what Mr. Johnson and his wife of forever needed in their golden years. I even thought about hospitalizing him to bring it under control but, luckily, came to my senses on this point.

I said, "Mr. Johnson, your blood pressure is very high, *very* high."

He'd been to a blood pressure screening van in a supermarket parking lot and been told that he should see a doctor. This probably saved his life.

"In fact, it's so high that I'm thinking that maybe you should go into the hospital."

He told me that he couldn't do that because he absolutely had to work to keep a dollar and a half ahead of his monthly expenses.

I said, "Okay, here's what I'm going to do. I'm going to start you on a blood pressure medicine and you have to come in to the clinic *every day* until your blood pressure is under control. That's the only other choice, and you better accept it before I change my mind and insist you go straight to the hospital."

Mr. Johnson was a big guy with a terrifically friendly face and big, bushy, gray eyebrows and little round wire-frame glasses that dated back to around 1940. He was a big, fuzzy, teddy bear kind of guy whom you wanted to give a great big hug. He was very straightforward and permanently perplexed by the medical business. He knew I was talking about big trouble but had no clear understanding of exactly how it all worked.

He scratched his head and spoke in his big, broad, open voice. "Gee, Doc. That bad, eh?"

I shook my head. "Worse."

Then he asked, "What is blood pressure anyway?"

I said, "Think of a heart as being a simple pump, just like any other kind of pump. Got that?"

He nodded.

I continued, "Well, every pump generates a certain amount of pressure, some more than others, right?"

132

He nodded again.

"And if the pressure gets too high, a pipe might burst, right?"

Another nod.

I said, "Well, you can think of it like that, although it gets a bit more complex inside of your body." I didn't tell him that this simple description fairly well summed up my own knowledge of the system, and to hell with the complexity. The system actually got very complex, involving not only the heart, but the blood vessels, the kidneys, and who knows what else. Some doctors even specialized in hypertension.

I shook my finger at him. "And, if one of the pipes that breaks is inside your head that means a big-time stroke and a great deal of major nonsense in the hospital with respirators and infections and bedsores. Understand?" I felt the need to scare him because his blood pressure was scaring me.

He scratched his head and nodded again. I sent him home with a prescription for blood pressure medicine and a promise to come back the next day. He did so, and in three weeks his BP was down to an absolutely incredibly normal 120/80. Some docs would even say that this was too low, that his body had acclimated to the higher pressure; but he had no problems at all.

Mr. Johnson came in every month like clockwork. I wrote out his prescription each time, and marked the paper to instruct the pharmacy to bill the clinic. This easily saved the patient $200 a month, an expense he would otherwise not be able to afford. I should add that there was literally no other way for Mr. Johnson to get his medicine, and that without the services of our clinic, he would certainly have had a stroke. Once this had happened, he'd have wound up slowly dying in the intensive care unit attached to a dozen machines. Once he was dead, the hospital would send his bill (ranging somewhere from a minimum of $50,000 to a max of, oh, around a half million, maybe more) to the Medicare administration, and they'd pay it. Our clinic, by creating a little tiny island of socialized medicine in a sea of fee-for-service, was actually using government money (in the form of our grant) to save government money. And providing good health care to boot. But don't tell that to a private doc—he might have a stroke.

Mr. Johnson and I had plenty of time left over after I'd refilled his meds, and I did all of the other "health maintenance," or preventive medicine, things that are supposed to be done for a guy his age. This included a chest X ray (which some would say is necessary and some would say isn't), testing the stool for blood (which everybody agrees is necessary), thorough physical, EKG, glaucoma screen (which everybody agrees is necessary but most forget to do), and so on.

I even asked him about sex. He was a little surprised. "Well, Doc, you know I'm not a young man anymore." I said, "So?"

He said, "So, things aren't as active as they used to be." I said, "Well, I don't want you to think that if you're not happy with your sex life that there's nothing to be done about it because you're getting old. The point is that you should be happy with however much sex you're having. Now, that's 'happy' and not 'accepting' or 'reconciled,' Okay?"

The idea that old age meant no sex was a major misconception that I tried to bring up with my older patients whenever I could. Some of them just refused to talk about it, but Mr. Johnson was so open and puzzled and straightforward that I figured I should push it with him. He wanted to know if there was a normal amount of sex for someone his age, and I told him that some was preferable to none, but that different people were happy with vastly different levels of some. What was important was happiness, not numbers. Mr. Johnson explained that he was happy, and I left it at that.

Mr. Johnson surprised me one day by bringing his wife in to meet me. She wore her Sunday best, and a big frilly hat just like Mrs. Sweet. She smiled broadly at me, like I was her favorite grandson. I was flattered and humbled.

I did give Mr. Johnson that big bear hug when I left the clinic, and handed his case over to one of the residents who was just starting. I assume that he still comes in every month to get his meds, just like clockwork, and still asks puzzled, straightforward questions.

Medicare legislation, by the way, has changed since Mr. Johnson was my patient. I'm not one hundred percent clear on the details, but I understand that Medicare will now pay for a percentage of the cost of outpatient meds, based on the patient's income. Whatever the system, I see it as an improvement. It will make critical meds available for millions of elderly people who, like big ol' Mr. Johnson, would otherwise not be able to afford them.

In New York State the issue of health insurance for "working poor" people under sixty-five years of age has also been addressed. Eligibility for Medicaid (the federal/state insurance program for the poor) has been expanded to include many of those whose incomes were previously not low enough for them to qualify. A family of six, for example, is now eligible with an income of $13,600 or less, up from $8,000. In other words, you now only have to be very poor, instead of rotten, stinking poor, to qualify. I'd like to see the administrators who run Medicaid support a family of *six* on thirteen grand. Still, it's a step in the right direction, and gives people an incentive to work.

Mrs. Guttierez was another of my favorites. I met her on the wards at NYG, where I treated her for pneumonia and subsequently stole her as a clinic patient. She was about eighty and didn't speak a word of English.

Possibly, I treated Mrs. Guttierez for something other than pneumonia. I don't remember exactly what she had, but do recall that it wasn't something too serious. People often get admitted to the hospital not because of extreme sickness, but because the ER doc is concerned they won't get good follow-up if they're sent home. Maybe Mrs. Guttierez was admitted out of concern that without close supervision her pneumonia would worsen and she'd decompensate and crash. A good ten or fifteen percent of the people we admitted fell into this category: lack of good outpatient care for illnesses that could be managed at home.

Some people didn't need admission at all and came into the hospital for "social" reasons, like old folks who'd been forgetting to take their medicines or leaving things on the stove and risked hurting themselves. "Social admissions" sometimes stayed in the hospital for months awaiting an appropriate "disposition." The lucky ones got a "home health aide," who'd cook, clean, shop (some even administered medications, though they weren't supposed to), and attend to other household chores so that the patient could remain at home. One patient might require a half-dozen services: visiting doctor, visiting nurse, home health aide, ambulance transport, social worker, and whatever else. Those who couldn't be managed at home awaited admission to a nursing home. These patients included the severely demented, the permanently bedridden, and those requiring twenty-four-hour nursing care.

One of my patients on the Cloud Pavilion had been awaiting a nursing home bed for months. In fact, as far as I could tell, she'd been waiting for years. I inherited her from the previous intern when I came on service, and when I looked in her chart I discovered that he'd also inherited her when he came on service. Her date of admission predated the earliest note in her chart (which was labeled "Volume 4 of 4 volumes"), and when I went down to the medical records office to look at her old records, they couldn't be found. Maybe she'd been on the Cloud Pavilion for decades.

She was a robust, physically intact, and moderately demented elderly lady, and every day the nurses hauled her out of bed, strapped her into a wheelchair, and deposited her in the hallway where she sang Yiddish songs at the top of her voice and grabbed at people's crotches as they walked by. I wrote a note in her chart every three days that read, "Progress unchanged. Await disposition." She was still up on Cloud when I finished my rotation, and I bequeathed her to the next intern. She may still be there today.

One middle-aged woman brought her two ancient and completely demented great-aunts into the ER at NYG, told me they had driven her nearly insane, and dumped them.

I said, "But you can't just leave them here! I mean, there's no medical reason to admit them!"

The woman said, "Doctor, I either leave them here or I go berserk."

I said, "How about if you talk to the social worker, and she'll start the process of getting them into a nursing home? It'll take a few weeks, max."

She said, "I won't last a few weeks. I'm sorry," and walked out.

While the two elderly ladies wandered around the ER mumbling to themselves, I asked the resident in charge of admissions what we should do. One woman walked in on a group of surgeons attending to a gunshot victim. She was gently escorted out of the surgical area of the ER and tied into a wheelchair.

I wound up admitting both women and have no idea what became of them.

"Disposition problems" were not limited to the elderly. One of my patients at NYG was a young woman with a skin infection that required a few days of intravenous antibiotics. When it was cured I told her that she was about to be discharged.

She said, "Where am I gonna go?"

I discovered that she didn't have a home or money. She'd walked into the ER off the street and had nowhere to go.

This seemed strange because she was young and fit and I wondered why, if she didn't work, she wasn't on welfare, staying with family, or whatever. Instead of discharging her I decided to keep her an extra day and have the social worker and shrink talk to her. They might have some ideas about what to do with her.

The shrink decided that the patient was crazy. This probably accounted for her being so unhinged from society. He also declared that the patient was competent (i.e., able to understand the consequences of her own actions), not a danger to herself or others, not psychotic (i.e., not completely disconnected from reality), and therefore not in need of psychiatric admission. The psych floor was always full, and trying to get a patient transferred there from a medical floor was literally impossible.

The social worker said she'd help the patient get onto welfare, but that it would take a while. I asked her if there was some . . . well . . . *place* the patient could go until then. As an intern I did not yet fully comprehend the world's cruelty. It seemed to me that there must be *something* to do for someone like that, some way to bridge the gap from being unconnected to being at least marginally connected. I was told that the patient could be given a subway token for getting to the women's shelter (naturally, this would require completing a form). That was it, a subway token and the women's shelter.

I asked my resident what to do. Maybe I should keep

the patient in the hospital until she got on welfare and hope that nobody noticed. If I did this, though, I'd at least need the approval of my immediate higher-up.

My resident gave me a long song and dance about being grown up and responsible for my own actions, and told me that the disposition of the patient was completely my own decision. She was a big liberal, too, and said, "I think you should decide on a responsible and caring disposition for this patient."

This pissed me off because I needed real guidance, and not a load of liberal claptrap rhetoric. A "responsible and caring disposition" did not appear to be possible. Still, I didn't want to antagonize my resident, so I sulked off on my own to decide what to do.

The next day I filled out the form to get the patient a subway token, gave her the address for the women's shelter and the phone number for the social worker, and discharged her. When we walked to her room on afternoon rounds my resident made a big stink when she saw that the patient was gone.

She said, "What did you do with her?"

I replied in a monotone, "I discharged her."

"Without checking with me?"

I was still sulking. "For what? You told me it was completely up to me what I did with her, and I decided to discharge her."

"What was her disposition?"

"A subway token, the address of the women's shelter, and the phone number of the social worker." In other words, I threw her out into the street.

She glared at me. "Was that all you could do?"

I glared back. "Sorry. I guess I should have married her." And then I walked out of the room.

Which is all to say that it pays to have someone who'll

take care of you. People became disposition problems when they didn't have anyone to look after them. Even a friend or a dedicated neighbor could be enough. One of my patients was an old gay man who'd lived in Harlem for something like fifty years. His lover had died many years before and, as his neighborhood deteriorated, he became terrified of going out. Eventually, he refused to go out at all, and his neighbor, a Hispanic woman and her children, took on the burden of looking after him.

He slowly began to develop congestive heart failure, but refused to see a doctor. Finally, his neighbor was forced to call an ambulance. I don't think he'd been out of his apartment in ten years when I saw him. He was in terrible shape, but also a tribute to how a little bit of help had enabled him to survive at home. He was a real misogynist, and refused to talk to any of the female staff, including my partner Dolores.

She was saddened and perplexed. She said, "I don't think that man likes women."

Eventually, we discharged him. I assume he is still in his apartment, a bent, sad recluse, surviving only through the generosity of his neighbor.

Mrs. Guttierez had dedicated family and friends galore. She was part of a tremendous extended Latino family filled with uncles and brothers and cousins, all of whom were totally devoted to her. The only thing that was missing was a doctor to manage her medical needs. The ER doc who admitted her probably would have sent her home if she'd had a community doc to provide follow-up. He'd call and say, "Hi, I'm Dr. So-and-so at the NYG ER. I'm seeing your patient, Mrs. Guttierez, who has pneumonia. I'm a little nervous about her, and I'd like to admit her, but I'd be willing to send her home if you agree to close follow-up." The only alternative was to send the patient to "medical clinic," which saw around a zillion patients daily, was a total zoo, and easily scared off the young and robust, never mind the old and frail. The ER doc who saw Mrs. Guttierez didn't think this was enough, so he admitted her to make sure she'd get thorough care. I was lucky to have her as a patient, and when I discharged her I gave her an appointment to come and see me at my own clinic office.

Mrs. Guttierez had several complex medical problems — heart failure, high blood pressure, asthma, and an abnormal heartbeat — and she came in frequently for the first few months to straighten them out one at a time. Although her family was dedicated, they worked during the day and could not stay at home to take care of her, so the clinic social worker arranged for her to have a home health aide. She and the patient fell in love immediately. At first, I thought she was a family member because she treated Mrs. Guttierez so sweetly.

The patient was a small, frail woman who sat silently during her appointments and refused to complain about anything. I asked my questions through the home health aide because I spoke almost no Spanish. "Please ask Mrs. Guttierez if anything in particular is bothering her today."

The home health aide would do so and the patient would mumble an inaudible response. "She says nothing bothers her."

I found her habit of playing the role of a demure and undemanding female to be frustrating and had to go through all of her problems one by one to make sure everything was okay. Then I'd spend fifteen minutes rewriting her dozen prescriptions, draw elaborate dose schedules, explain everything several times to the aide, and finally send her home.

One day Mrs. Guttierez came in without an appointment, complaining of fever and cough. That is, she was dragged in by the aide, and forced to admit that she was sick. I examined her and took an X ray and discovered she again had pneumonia.

141

Had I been in the emergency room, I would simply have admitted her. The combination of age, frailty, and sickness added up to an appropriate admission. In the clinic, however, I could use myself to provide the needed follow-up and manage her at home with her family. I called the home health aide and an accompanying family member into my tiny office to explain the options.

I said, "Mrs. Guttierez has pneumonia." They groaned in unison. "Now, there's two things we can do. I can give you a prescription for medicine to take at home, but you have to watch her like a hawk and keep in close touch with me by phone and bring her back tomorrow afternoon so I can see how she's doing, or I can put her in the hospital."

Mrs. Guttierez's home health aide and family member loved her and decided to keep her at home. I gave them a prescription for penicillin and told them all of the bad signs to look for that would necessitate hospitalization (high fever, inability to take anything by mouth, and increasing lethargy).

I called later that night and the next morning. Her family had taken her temperature every two hours during the night, recorded everything she'd eaten, and described her condition as though they were professional nurses. She came back to the clinic in the afternoon looking just a little bit better (this was all in my mind because the pneumonia would require at least thirty-six hours to show a response), and the next day looking even better, and two days later looking almost cured. A repeat X ray showed that the pneumonia had shrunk considerably. A week later she was completely back to normal.

Mrs. Guttierez was a real success. Her family and I kept her out of the hospital.

I don't even remember the name of one of my other

successes, a man who walked into the ER, stopped breathing, and collapsed. He was a middle-aged guy who'd just been at a friend's house for dinner, started to feel bad, and drove himself to the hospital. Just in time, too, because he stopped breathing right after I asked him, "What's the matter?"

I stuck an intubation tube in his throat and attached him to a respirator. He turned from an awful shade of oxygenless ashy blue to pink in about five minutes. His family came in about a half hour later and went in to see him before I had a chance to talk to them. This is always a bad idea when your relative has a big ugly tube sticking out of his mouth and is attached to a machine and can't talk.

They came back out looking horrified. He had one son, a fellow about twenty-three years old who was an ambulance tech, who grilled me about why I'd tubed his old man.

He said, "Was my father cyanotic, Doctor?" I imagined myself in his position and decided he was probably feeling sad and terrified and also like he needed to take some control of the situation. This would explain his use of medical jargon. I didn't want to be patronizing because this seemed a reasonable response to what had happened.

I said, "I know this has to be really terrible for you, but I really absolutely had to intubate your father; he stopped breathing right in front of me. There was nothing else to do."

The son slumped over a little and stopped trying to bluster. He said, "He did?"

I said, "Yeah, but I really do think he's going to do well, I really do. He's going to do fine." This was based more on a gut feeling than anything else, but it was the truth about how I felt.

The amazing thing about the whole episode was that I really did save the guy's life and, contrary to the conservation of malignancy theory, not only was he a good guy, but he did fine. I went to visit him a few days later on the ward and he was sitting with his wife and two kids talking. Much better than they should be at his funeral. It felt really good, it was one of those moments when being a doctor felt terrific, like it made a hell of a difference.

There was another patient, a big, heavy older woman who'd been battling with an asthma attack for days and days, and finally came into the ER because she was getting too damn tired to breathe. I gave her all the routine medications but she got worse and worse and more and more exhausted.

Finally she started to look like she would soon stop breathing and I'd have to intubate her and use a respirator. I was worried about this because she was big and fat and strong and awake and terrified. There'd be a horrible scene with a lot of snot flying around and struggling and yelling, "Suction!! Where the hell is the goddam suction!?" You had to have suction when you intubated someone to suck out all the saliva and snot and vomit and blood that got in the way of seeing where to put the tube. As I said earlier, it's much easier to tube someone who is dead. Dead people don't fight or require explanations.

The head nurse was a friend of mine. She'd even given me a ride home once, and introduced me to her crazy brother and sister, who'd come to the hospital to pick her up at the end of her shift.

She was helping me tend to the patient and I kept asking her, "Jeez, this lady is starting to look shitty . . . whaddaya think . . . huh, think I oughta tube her, or what?"

She had no compunctions about talking to me normally.

She said, "Listen, I can't make the decision for you, but I think you should go with your gut feelings on this one." She knew my gut feelings were saying, "For Christ's sake, tube her now before she kicks the bucket."

So, I intubated her. It turned out that she was so exhausted from trying to breathe that she barely fought at all. I sprayed her throat with local anesthetic and talked her through it and got the tube into her trachea with no problem.

It wasn't until she started to get enough oxygen to move around that she started fighting. I didn't want her to pull the tube out so I pumped her full of Valium to make her calm down.

It was naturally at the moment that she finally fell asleep, looking like a big, pale, beached walrus in some sort of bizarre medical experiment, that her extremely well-educated adult daughter came in, took one look at her, and started making a very big stink.

"Where is the goddam doctor that did this to my mother?!"

She was understandably upset. It has to be difficult to get a phone call saying, "Mom's in the hospital, get down there as soon as possible," and to jump in a cab and come bursting into the ER all out of breath and discover your half-naked mother lying comatose on a stretcher attached to this ugly, hissing machine, apparently more than a little bit sick.

I spent a half hour explaining all the medical reasons why she needed to be tubed. There were a series of blood values that could be used to make the decision to intubate a patient, and I'd actually had the presence of mind to get them before I'd done so, so that I could put them in her chart. I used these values to demonstrate to the patient's daughter that her mom had to be treated the way she was. This calmed her down a bit. I never said, "Look, your mom looked like shit, she couldn't breathe, so I went with my gut and tubed her," which is what happened, and which is what almost always happens when a patient is intubated on an emergency basis, regardless of the blood values.

145

When I went to check on the patient a few days later she was sitting up, no tube, surrounded by beaming family. They all greeted me warmly and effused thanks, even the ornery one, who took me aside and said, "I'm really sorry I gave you so much trouble. I can see that you saved my mother's life. Thanks."

I played the role of mature, professional type and puffed up my chest, saying, "That's perfectly okay. It's your right to ask as many questions as you want. I'd consider it abnormal for you not to get upset in a situation like that." What I wanted to say was, "Yeah, well, don't worry about it, though you can get really bitchy, can't you?!"

About three or four months later the educated young daughter came in for a minor problem and was seen by one of the other docs. I recognized her although I didn't remember where from, and said, "I know you."

She looked at me for a long moment and said, "I've thought about you many times, Doctor. You saved my mother's life." There was something both sultry and serious in her voice.

I wanted to say, "That's right, you're the ornery, bitchy, good-looking daughter of that lady I tubed. Got any ideas about how you'd like to demonstrate your gratitude?"

Instead, naturally, I started to get nervous and blurted, "Oh, yeah! How's she doing?"

She looked at me for another long moment and replied, "She's doing fine, Doctor, thank you."

Not only was that one of the few moments where I felt halfway deserving of my medical degree, but I almost asked her out to dinner.

8

Lethal Hospitals,
Deadly Doctors

My experience with Uncle Melvin, Mr. Smith, Mr. Cloud, and just about all the rest of my patients taught me that hospitals were not such good places for sick people. In fact, they were extraordinarily dangerous places, much more suited to the strong and robust than the sick and debilitated. Hazards lurked everywhere: incompetent and overaggressive attendings, fatigued housestaff, pissed-off nurses, apathetic ancillary staff. The reality of doctor-induced illness was so much a part of medicine that there was a word for it: "iatrogenic." Even the hospital building, the physical facility itself, could be dangerous, as though it had an evil Stephen King-like presence. This condition was described by the word "nosocomial." Iatrogenic and nosocomial illnesses are both subjects that I would like to discuss at length.

Nosocomial illness was most often the result of the various species of killer bacteria that set up housekeeping within a hospital's walls. Battle-hardened microbes, made immune to multiple assaults with toxic and expensive medications by a roguish capacity to mutate, lurked everywhere, and assaulted the innocent patient at random and without warning. In the usual scenario, the patient appeared to be doing quite well and then suddenly "spiked a temp." In the surgical patient this meant that a commando bacteria had found its way into the operative wound and, in an orgy of nonsexual replication, established an entire population of its mutant offspring. Brilliantly colorful and distinctively pungent infections developed overnight.

The patient entombed on the medical ward whose immune defenses were weakened by illness provided other gateways of infection. Typically, the lungs were the first site of infestation, followed by the bladder, the kidneys, and the bedsores. Grotesque and complicated infections fascinated the housestaff, who immediately called the bug docs for consultation. These specialists traveled in caravans, and arrived trailing long white coats, freshly scrubbed medical students, very concerned social service workers, culture dishes, test tubes, needles and syringes, gloves, gowns, masks, and a formidable array of the absolute latest experimental treatments.

Bug docs, incidentally, were the only specialists to use the sense of smell in diagnosis, often identifying the bacteria causing an infection by its particular odor. Although putting one's nose within vomiting distance of an infected wound might give the average person second thoughts, I considered this quality a commendable one.

A favorite prof in medical school was a bug doc who lectured on the scent of different critters. He'd sit in front of the class wearing a baseball cap, an array of different culture dishes laid out before him. One of the students would then blindfold him and hold a dish under his nose.

He'd sniff, pause, and sniff again. "Hmm, yes . . . yes, that's a 'seventy-eight pseudomonas, I can tell by that fine sweet lingering aroma. A particularly virulent year." He was rarely wrong.

Once, while working in the NYG emergency room, I examined a fifteen-year-old girl who had pelvic inflammatory disease, a sexually transmitted infection of the uterus. When the patient got up in the stirrups for a pelvic exam, a nauseating odor of infection came wafting up out of her crotch. Just the smell was enough to let me know she needed to stay in the hospital. When I finished the exam I told her she needed to be admitted, but she became resistant. Nothing I could say would change her mind.

Finally, I pretended to give up. "Well, I guess if you want to go home with your vagina smelling like this, there's really nothing I can do about it." I waved the used speculum under her nose.

She agreed immediately to be admitted.

In Australia several years ago there was a hospital outbreak of a bug called MRSA, methicillin resistant staph aureus. Staph (short for "staphylococcus") aureus is a bug with a particular proclivity to develop resistance to the antibiotics used against it. At one time it was easily eradicated with penicillin but, after a few decades, it became almost uniformly resistant. Methicillin, a semisynthetic penicillin, was then discovered, and this problem was solved. The bacterium continued the game of cat and mouse by then developing resistance to methicillin. The first strains of MRSA emerged in Australia.

One of the Australian doctors at the stricken hospital was interviewed on public television (one of my major sources of medical information). He discussed the mechanisms by which bacteria become drug resistant. The usual cause is indiscriminate antibiotic use, the frequent switching from one drug to the next in an infected patient. When the dose of the drug is too low, or the duration of use too short, the infection is subdued rather than eradicated. There are zillions of bugs in even the smallest infection, and when the infection simmers, many generations of bacteria are produced. This creates ideal conditions for Darwinian natural selection, the production and refinement of chance genetic mutations that allow a species to survive a given stress. In this case, the species is whatever type of bacteria is causing the infection, and the stress is the action of the antibiotic. One mechanism of resistance, for example, is the development of an enzyme that enables the bacteria to break down the antibiotic molecule, rendering it ineffective (this was

149

how penicillin resistance first arose). Another is the production of a barrier to the drug's penetration of the bacterial cell wall. Whatever the method, the nonresistant bacteria die off, and the resistant bacteria produce a whole new population. When doctors piss around with a little bit of antibiotic here and a little bit there, the end result is Rambo bacteria that have seen and survived it all.

The Australian doc was particularly critical of the class of antibiotics called cephalosporins, "broad spectrum" drugs that kill a wide variety of organisms. He believed that infections are best treated by identifying the causative organism and destroying it with a drug of known effectiveness. Broad-spectrum drugs fit in with more of a shotgun approach to treating infection. Using a drug that kills a broad spectrum of bacteria is easier than identifying one bug in particular (even if it is only an educated guess), and using an antibiotic with more specific action. The doc on the program called cephalosporins "the wasteland of the diagnostically destitute." He'd even started a newsletter devoted to the subject of inappropriate antibiotic use.

I don't remember what happened to MRSA in Australia. Perhaps they had to burn down the hospital and shoot all of the infected patients to keep it from spreading. In the United States MRSA is now fairly common, and there are relatively new drugs used to kill it. I assume that staph will eventually develop resistance to these drugs, and then we too will have to burn down our hospitals and shoot all of our patients. I can't wait.

Bacterial guerrilla warfare is the least of the problems inherent to the hospital. The staff itself is by far the single greatest danger within its walls, with doctors, nurses, and related medical staff injuring and killing patients regularly and unavoidably. Iatrogenic injury is, in fact, so common, and often so interesting, that I've thought of founding an "American Journal of Iatrogenics," to document the folly for all to enjoy.

Incompetence, indifference, insanity, and the simple commission of error are normal elements of the human condition. That they run amok in the medical profession, killing and maiming innocent people, should come as little surprise. The same is true of other professions, and the relative import of their outcome is a matter of opinion. A doctor screws up and kills a patient, a general screws up and kills a battalion, a bureaucrat screws up and deprives a widow of her pension. Who's to say which is worse?

Regardless of the commonality of catastrophe, the medical profession has long enjoyed a reputation of learned infallibility. True, it has recently come under a more critical public eye, and the erstwhile reverence of doctors as godlike is long gone. In fact, medicine is increasingly on the defensive. Lawyers solicit malpractice suits in television commercials and advanced medical technology is castigated as "inhumane" on talk shows and news specials. Still, the extent of the problem, the degree to which ineptitude, apathy, and outright lunacy create bad medical practice is little known to the public in general.

Occasionally, once every few years, some poor, hapless, sleep-deprived intern accidentally offs a famous person. Usually it's no big deal, maybe an unforeseen drug allergy or side effect, but, lo and behold, the hospital finds itself saddled with a celebrity cadaver. A big stink follows, reviews are convened, recommendations made, the intern and an attending or two are ceremonially sacrificed, and then the whole thing blows over. Human error, however, is not prevented by reviews, recommendations, or sacrifices, and the cycle is inevitably repeated, whether it's days, months, or years later, providing more fodder for the tabloids. All the while everyday folks are being knocked off in hospitals the world over every day of the year. It is a fact of life, or perhaps a fact of death, and it shouldn't surprise anyone because it isn't possible not to make mistakes.

I've made my share of mistakes, though through the

grace of fortune, or providence, never killed anyone. One such episode involved an ancient woman whom I was treating for asthma on one of the medical wards at NYG, early on in my internship year.

Asthma, a truly brutal disease, involves narrowing and obstruction of the airways, the tiny tubes that lead air deep down into the lungs. This is caused by a buildup of mucus within the airways, and spasm of the tiny muscular coats that surround them. In a moderate asthma attack, the patient experiences little trouble inhaling because the airways are widened as the chest expands, making it easier for air to pass through them. On exhalation, however, the chest contracts and the airways are narrowed. This compounds the blockage that already exists and severely reduces air flow. The patient must exhale forcibly, and the high-velocity movement of air through the narrowed passages makes a high-pitched wheezing sound that can be heard with a stethoscope. When an attack is severe, air flow is restricted during both inhalation and exhalation, and the wheezing of the struggling patient is plainly audible. Treatment of asthma is directed at widening the airways and clearing the mucus buildup so that breathing becomes easier.

Asthma is a particularly vicious disease in that it strikes early as well as late in life, the smoker as well as the non-smoker, those who attend to their health as well as those who do not. It is a disease without reason, a chronic disease that rarely kills, but robs people of their ability to be productive and lead normal lives.

Most asthmatic patients are treated in the emergency room using a combination of inhaled and injected medications. If an attack does not "break" within a few hours the patient is admitted for further treatment and observation. It's a bad idea to send someone home who is having difficulty breathing. My patient, a ninety-five-year-old woman, had begun to breathe much easier after a few days of therapy when she quite suddenly became very tight. A nurse paged to tell me she was having difficulty, and I hurried to her bedside to find her gasping and sputtering for air. She became progressively worse despite a series of inhalation treatments and injections, and soon started to tire from the effort of breathing. Finally, she turned a rotten shade of blue, threw in the towel, and stopped breathing altogether.

Incredibly, I'd foreseen this possibility and had an intubation tray at the ready. I calmly tubed the patient and attached her to a respirator to do her breathing for her. Once the tube was in and the machine doing an adequate job of providing her with oxygen, she turned pink, perked right up, and demonstrated her gratitude by thrashing wildly about on the bed. The tube and machine, though doing a much better job of breathing for her than she had been able to do on her own, also caused a paradoxical sense of choking. I grabbed her hand and begged her to calm down, explaining that relaxing and allowing the machine to work would stop the terrifying feeling of air hunger. Suffocation, however, does not reconcile a patient to reason. The woman completely ignored me, stared wildly around the room with terrified eyes, got more and more agitated, knocked over the bedside table, and tried repeatedly to rip the tube out of her throat.

The next logical step would be sedation. The humanist approach wasn't working, the room was rapidly becoming a shambles, and I was breaking into a sweat restraining a berserk ninety-five-year-old woman. A quick squirt of Valium or Demerol would quiet things down nicely and remove any concern of the patient extubating herself (removing the tube) and dying. Valium would be a good choice for a younger person, but sometimes caused increased agitation in the elderly. It also had the potential to drop the patient's blood pressure and calm her down permanently. Demerol, a narcotic painkiller and sedative related to morphine and heroin, seemed the best alternative. It too might lower her blood pressure, but its effects could be reversed with naloxone, the miracle drug I'd used so successfully to wake up sleepy junkies in the ER.

153

I filled a syringe with 50 mg of Demerol and slowly squeezed half into the IV in the patient's arm. Intravenous Demerol works remarkably quickly, and the patient calmed visibly within thirty seconds. Still, she was not calm enough. She continued to flail about on the bed and make sporadic attempts to pull out the tube.

Next came the bad part, the part where I failed to carefully consider my actions in the manner that, so far, had worked so well. My next move was a perfect example of the kind of unthinking action that kills people.

I decided, "What the hell, I'll just give her the rest," and emptied the syringe into the IV.

It had the desired effect. The patient ceased flailing and flopped down in bed. For good measure I checked her pulse, which seemed quite strong, and proceeded to write a note in her chart for the staff in the intensive care unit. Hospital policy dictated that all asthmatic patients who got tubed were transferred to the ICU.

I wrote a brief description of the patient's hospital course and physical exam, but hestitated before recording her vital signs (blood pressure, temperature, pulse, and respirations). The most recent vitals had been taken by the nurse several hours earlier. I knew they should be rechecked after all the excitement, but wasn't in the mood to drag my ass out of my chair and hunt down a blood pressure cuff. Too much hassle. It'd be much easier just to make them up. Besides, the patient would be in the ICU in less than a half hour, and she would get a complete physical soon after she arrived. I made up a new set of vitals and recorded them in her chart. When I finished I stood up and walked to her bedside. She was still lying quietly. I turned and walked out of the room.

Every halfway decent doc's brain has a part set aside for what I like to think of as a panel of little red lights. Each red light corresponds to a specific medical scenario, and automatically goes on when that scenario is encountered. The doc sees the red light go on, and understands its meaning:

154

If the patient is not attended to diligently and properly, he will become either critically ill or dead. It's not really important whether the patient lives or dies, but that appropriate care be given. In my mind, the brightest little red light is the one labeled, "Patient is short of breath!!" In fact, this was the red light that brought me running into the current patient's room to begin with. When I see it go on I understand that I must see to it that everything possible is done to prevent the patient's deterioration or that someone else (say, the ICU doc) assumes this responsibility. Death is not the preferred outcome, but acceptable if I've done everything possible. If, on the other hand, the patient deteriorates or dies and I haven't done everything possible, that is very, very bad. It is cause for losing my license.

I'd gotten two steps past the patient's room when several red lights went on in my head simultaneously. One said, "This patient is critically ill!!" Another said, "At this moment, you, and no one else, are solely responsible for this critically ill patient's life!!" Another said, "Critically ill patients can deteriorate rapidly!!" The brightest light was flashing frantically. It said, "Lying is bad medicine!!!"

I turned around and walked back into the patient's room to take her vital signs. I discovered that the poor old woman's blood pressure was down around 40, making her ripe for transfer from NYG to the ninth floor over on the Cloud Pavilion.

I ran to the nurses' station, filled a syringe with a bunch of naloxone, ran back to the patient's bedside, and squirted it into her IV. She bounded back up in the bed and resumed flailing about and knocking things over. I rechecked her blood pressure. It had returned to a healthy 100. Thank God for little red lights.

The patient was transferred to the ICU where she did well. The tube came out of her throat a few days later and she was discharged within a week.

That was the closest I ever came to accidentally killing anyone in the hospital.

* * *

Another of my iatrogenic episodes involved an alcoholic junkie in the NYG emergency room. This patient, like Miss Davis, the junkie, transvestite hooker with AIDS, had been a big-time addict for years and had scarred over all his veins from his needle habit. For this reason, he also needed one of those big, nasty, central lines in his neck, so that we'd be able to take blood tests and give him medicine.

The process of placing a central line is the closest a medical doctor ever gets to a surgical procedure. A gigantic pencil-sized needle is repeatedly thrust into the patient's neck, like a deranged sewing machine, until it hits the internal jugular (IJ) vein, a tremendous blood vessel that carries blood draining from the head. The needle has a wide bore and, once it's in, a catheter is fed through it into the vein. The needle is then pulled out and slipped off the end of the catheter, which is attached to an IV line and sewed to the skin to hold it in place.

A central line is the ideal labor-saving device for interns dealing with veinless junkies. It provides access for removing blood or for administering medication and lasts much longer than the average IV, which is supposed to be changed every forty-eight hours. At MH, the interns were supposed to replace central lines every three days because of the risk of infection, but we generally left them in until our residents yelled at us to change them.

Sometimes junkies themselves catch on to the idea of a central line and, after getting out of the hospital, stick dirty needles into their own necks in search of the IJ to shoot in junk. Unfortunately for the junkie or anyone else who goes prodding about in people's necks with large gauge needles, there is a very large artery just beneath the IJ, called the carotid. This is easily stabbed and, even nicked, bleeds like the proverbial stuck pig. It wasn't until I became an intern that I learned the expression "going for the jugular" would more appropriately be "going for the carotid." The presence of the carotid makes life all the much more exciting for the enterprising junkie. He is adding the sixth and final bullet to the revolver, placing it to his temple, and pulling the trigger.

I'd never hit the carotid before, but on that day in the ER I did. It was easy to tell because as soon as the needle struck a blood vessel and I removed the syringe to feed in the catheter, bright red arterial blood spurt out all over my shirt. This taught me, if nothing else, to always wear a gown while placing a central line.

Though poking the carotid is not considered good form, the bleeding is easily stopped by applying pressure to the side of the patient's neck. Resigning myself to practicality, if not perfect technique, I took some blood from the inadvertently punctured artery for routine lab tests, removed the needle, leaned on the patient's neck for a few minutes, and left the central line to be tried again another time. About a half hour later I checked the labs, one of which was a "coagulation profile." Its result was grossly abnormal; the patient's blood had lost most of its capacity to clot. This, probably, was the result of alcohol-induced liver disease.

After a moment or two of thought I realized that nonclotting blood plus a hole in a major artery might add up to a bit of trouble, and wandered back to the patient's bedside to have a look-see. When I lifted up the sheet, I discovered a grapefruit-sized mass right at the spot where I'd been sticking the patient with needles. With a little squeeze I could make blood come spouting out of the hole in his skin like a tiny, red fountain. The patient, who was now comfortably asleep, did not seem any the worse. I decided that the pressure of the blood itself would prevent any further bleeding and went back to my work without mucking about further, an action that would probably only have made things worse.

The patient did wind up dying, though not of causes related to this episode. Perhaps someone else killed him.

The fact that doctors are faulted for making an occasional honest (if deadly) mistake is unfortunate. Mistakes cannot

157

be prevented and there are deeper and more important problems in medicine that result in dishonest mistakes, like incompetence, indifference, and insanity. These issues, which I alluded to earlier, are characteristics all too common among medical people.

One evening a friend who was a supervising resident at NYG admitted a young man with pneumonia.

He told me, "This was a young guy like around twenty-five. A nice guy, too, not a junkie or a burglar." We tended to get condescending about junkies because so many of them were scumbags. Most of us tried not to let our condescending attitudes affect the way we treated patients. Sometimes we were successful.

My friend's patient was the average low-risk patient with pneumonia. He wasn't a junkie or a drinker, two factors that would put him at much higher risk of dying from pneumonia. He was admitted because he'd been vomiting and was unable to hold down oral medications, so he had to get the antibiotics intravenously.

On the initial chest X ray there was a hazy area in his lungs, indicating the pneumonia, and a pleural effusion. "Pleural effusion" is medical lingo for fluid around the lungs. Sometimes people with pneumonia get a collection of fluid at the base of the lung, which can be seen on the X ray. If the X ray is taken with the person standing up, what is called an air-fluid level is seen at the base of the lung. This means you can see the fluid, and you can see the air over the fluid, too. Computer people would say it was possible to see the "interface" between air and fluid. That the fluid is freely moving and has collected in the space around the lungs is confirmed by taking a second chest X ray while the patient is lying on his side. In accordance with gravity the fluid "layers out" along the sides of the lungs rather than at the bases. Such sideways chest X rays are called lateral decubitus views.

I'm not sure why people with pneumonia sometimes get pleural effusions, and my friend wasn't either.

He said, "I figured people with pneumonia just sometimes get effusions and if we treated him with antibiotics it would probably go away in a few days, but I called the lung docs just to make sure."

The lung docs showed up in their long white coats with a gaggle of residents and medical students. They peered intensely at the X rays, examined the patient, peered at the X rays again, held a conference, and returned with the verdict.

"Well, patients with pneumonia sometimes get pleural effusions. Treat him with antibiotics for a few days and call us if it doesn't go away."

The patient was treated with antibiotics for a few days and got much better but the effusion didn't go away.

My friend said, "This guy looked like shit when he came in and after two days of penicillin he looked a million percent better. We'd go into his room on rounds and he'd say, 'Hey, Doc! How you doing? I feel great, Doc. When do I get out of this joint?' And he really did, he looked great."

Still, my friend didn't feel right about discharging the patient with a pleural effusion. So, he decided to needle it and make sure everything was okay.

Normally, each lung is covered with a slippery, slimy layer of tissue called the pleura. The inner surface of the chest cavity is also covered by a layer of pleura, and the two layers slip and slide over each other as the lungs expand and contract in the normal process of breathing. Usually, there is nothing between these two layers, in the "pleural space," but a few ounces of lubricating juice. When a patient develops a pleural effusion, the pleural space fills up with fluid and the adjacent lung begins to collapse. "Needling" (intern's slang for thoracentesis, or "chest tap") a pleural effusion involves sticking a needle in between two ribs at the base of the patient's lung into the pleural space, and sucking out some of the pleural effusion juice. The fluid is then sent to the lab where it is scrutinized under microscopes and prodded mercilessly to make sure it is not dangerous.

Sometimes people have gigantic pleural effusions filling up half or three quarters of their lungs. These patients undergo "therapeutic" chest taps to remove fluid so they can breathe better. One of the patients at NYG was a lady with lung cancer who'd get a tremendous pleural effusion about twice a month and come into the emergency room short of breath and foaming at the mouth. The tumor in her lung behaved just like a leaky faucet. It dripped and dripped and dripped fluid that built up until it had taken up just about all the space in her chest and she couldn't breathe. Whoever was on call went down to the emergency room, stuck a needle into her back, and drained off a few liters of fluid. She then felt much better, although she eventually died of the cancer. It was terrific to be the one to needle her because it actually made her feel better. Making someone actually feel better was a much rarer occasion in the hospital than I'd believed before I went into medicine.

My friend needled the patient but was unable to get any fluid. He called the lung docs and they came flourishing back armed with a wide array of needles, but they also were unable to get any fluid. Assuming that everyone had done the most possible for the patient, my friend planned on discharging him the following day.

Unfortunately, he underestimated the wrath of a specialist scorned. The lung doc fellow, Dr. Lung, Jr. (the guy doing a lung doc fellowship, a one-year training period when he'd learn all the details about lungs) refused to believe that he could not get any fluid, and, after getting permission from his boss, Dr. Lung, Sr., took the patient to try the tap under fluoro.

In fluoroscopy ("fluoro") a big X-ray screen is put in front of the patient and turned on, bathing everyone in the room in green light and low-level radiation. The doc, who wears a lead-lined apron to protect himself from the radiation, can see all of the patient's gizzards in action on the screen. The difference between an X ray and fluoro is like the difference between a still photo and a movie.

Dr. Lung, Jr., wheeled the patient into the fluoro room and placed him behind the screen. The pleural effusion juice was easily visible, tantalizingly close, and he aimed the needle right at it. He stuck the patient six or seven or maybe ten times, but still didn't get any fluid.

Sighing, he glanced at his watch. It was almost four-thirty in the afternoon! He piled the patient back in the wheelchair, rushed him back to his room, and hurtled out of the hospital. He would try the tap again the following morning.

It was a good thing my friend was on the compulsive side and kept a close eye on his hospitalized patients. He rounded with his interns at about eleven o'clock the same night. They found the pneumonia patient lying in bed looking very pale and sweaty. This was surprising because he'd looked pretty good the same afternoon.

My friend asked him, "What's the matter?"

He replied, "Gee, I don't know, Doc. Ever since those guys took me downstairs and tried to take the fluid this afternoon I've been feeling lousy."

My friend said, "What guys? What downstairs?"

The patient replied, "You know, those lung doctor guys, they took me to that big X-ray machine and tried to get out some of that fluid in my lung."

My friend examined the patient. His belly was hard and tender and his blood pressure dangerously low. He called the surgeons, who came and took one look at him before wheeling him off to the operating room. When they opened up his belly they found a half-dozen holes in his spleen and about a liter of blood in his abdominal cavity.

Dr. Lung, Jr., had been a bit overeager when he tapped the patient under fluoro. He'd stuck the needle right through the pleural space into the upper part of the abdominal cavity, puncturing his spleen. The spleen is a very vascular organ and, given another hour, the patient would have

161

bled to death. My friend and the surgeons saved the patient's life. The surgeons removed his spleen, stopped the bleeding, and closed his abdomen.

My friend, who had a terrific temper when he got mad, called the lung doc fellow at home at 4:00 A.M. when the patient got out of the OR.

He said, "Hello, this is Dr. Resident at NYG. I understand you took my patient downstairs yesterday afternoon and did a chest tap under fluoro on him without my permission."

Dr. Lung, Jr., made an attempt to get huffy. "I really don't think it's necessary to call at four in the morn—"

My friend cut in, "I don't give two shits what you do or don't think is necessary. All you need to do is give me a good, clear explanation of why you didn't check with me before doing a procedure on my patient."

The fellow began the Nuremberg defense. "Listen, if you have a problem with this perhaps you should speak to Dr. Lung, Sr., because he was the one who gave me permission to attempt the tap under fluoro—"

My friend interrupted again, "I think I will. I think I'll call him right this very second. And I think I'll tell him that you put six holes in my patient's spleen and that he had a liter of blood in his belly when they opened him up in the OR two hours ago."

Then he hung up and called Dr. Lung, Sr., who was also in bed asleep. He said, "Dr. Lung, this is Dr. Resident. I'm on call over at NYG. Young Dr. Lung, Jr., asked me to make sure I called you to register a complaint."

The big-cheese lung doc got out an indignant, attending-level, who-the-hell-does-this-dirtball-resident-think-he-is-waking-me-up-in-the-middle-of-the-night-sounding snort and said, "Now, young man, it's four-fifteen in the morn—"

My friend, who at forty was the oldest resident in the hospital and also older than Dr. Lung, Sr., cut him off. He was neither enamored of nor impressed by his superiors in the hospital.

"I'm well aware of the time, thank you, Dr. Lung. Now, as I was saying, it seems that you asked Dr. Lung, Jr., to take my patient to do a chest tap under fluoro today. I'll be sure to inform Dr. Big that you did this without my permission or knowledge and that your flunkey put six holes in the patient's spleen that sent him to the OR. I'll be sure and tell Dr. Big that since we had no idea the patient had been retapped it was pure luck that we were on call and discovered him lying in bed bleeding into his abdomen at eleven P.M. rather than dead in his bed at eight A.M. Good night, Dr. Lung, you can go back to sleep now. Sorry to wake you."

He then called Dr. Big and told him the story. I fear to think of what became of the Drs. Lung.

I like this tale not only because it demonstrates that I'm not the only one who has made near catastrophic mistakes on patients but also because my pal's temper was so righteous and terrific. It is, in fact, a chilling example of a very common form of patient abuse in the hospital, one much worse than the accidental slip of a knife or an uncharacteristic and rare careless thought.

It is an example of the kind of thing that happens when docs cease to think of patients as people but instead see them as disease entities, organ systems from which they can gain experience in procedures that are not always medically necessary. By looking at patients in this way it is not too difficult to forget about the planning, the coordination, the care, and the thinking twice that is called for in treating a patient who is, after all, someone's brother, sister, father, mother, son, or daughter. The thinking, conscious or not, becomes, "We'll whip the guy downstairs, tap his chest, get a whole bunch of teaching and fun out of it, and be home before five." What it really should be is, "Does the guy really need his chest tapped? Does he understand why it needs to be done? Will it be dangerous to do to him? If he gets into trouble have we assured he'll be attended to? Are we doing this for his benefit or for our benefit?" And, of course, "Will we be home before five anyhow?"

163

When docs don't care they don't ask these questions. They don't believe, or have forgotten somewhere along the way, that these are the most important questions to ask, that forgetting to ask them constitutes bad medical practice. That, in fact, completing a medical procedure with perfect technical skill but without considering these questions is almost as bad as physically injuring the patient. In some ways it is worse because it reinforces the doc's belief that he can cruise merrily along without ever stopping to think about what he's doing. That his patients fail to suffer serious physical injury is merely a matter of luck. Luck always changes, and the patients of docs who don't care, who are burned out and don't take the time to sit down and think, will inevitably suffer more harm than good.

9

On Sunday the Doctors
Stayed Home

I had a clinic patient who died of plain old neglect and carelessness during an admission at Manhattan Hospital. He was one of my favorite patients and I saw him regularly at my clinic office. He was both a homosexual and a junkie, a double whammy in the 1980s, and supported himself and his habit by ripping off clothing stores, an occupation that he described to me in great detail. I believed him because he was a very snappy dresser. He fell into the category of patients that medical people would refer to as "dirtballs" or "scumbags," both by virtue of being a junkie and a criminal.

Nonetheless, I liked him a lot. He had AIDS-Related Complex, or ARC, a syndrome comprised of infection with the AIDS virus (HIV), lymphadenopathy (swollen lymph nodes), and oral thrush (yeast in the mouth). He had yet to develop the kind of major "opportunistic" infection that would put him in the category of full-blown AIDS. On his clinic visits I'd examine him and draw his blood (carefully), and he'd give me a hug before he left the office, saying, "Thanks and God bless you, Mr. Intern." For some reason he always called me "Mr." instead of "Dr." I first met him at NYG, when I was his intern during one of his admissions, and I remained his doc for the rest of the three years of my medical training. On his last visit at the clinic before I finished my training, he gave me a beautiful wood-encased desk clock that I still keep at home.

Every time he developed coughing, fever, or vomiting, Mr. Martinez had to be admitted to the hospital to make sure he didn't have a big-time infection. Whenever he felt bad he'd come to see me at the clinic, and I'd arrange for him to go to the hospital where he'd be cultured and X-rayed from head to toe. Then, once the cultures and X rays failed to show anything seriously wrong, he'd be sent home. This happened three or four times while I was his doctor and, so far, all the admissions had been false alarms.

Mr. Martinez got sick one Thursday evening about six months after I left MH. His case had been taken over by one of my co-workers, but the clinic had already closed for the day by the time he started to feel ill. Feverish and vomiting, he had no choice but to trundle off to the emergency room to be admitted. He took a cab to the ER and, after a brief exam by a resident and several hours of waiting, was finally shipped up to one of the wards. Unfortunately, no one attempted to get in touch with his clinic doc to let him know he was being admitted. Not only would this have been polite, but it would have allowed his doc to check in over the weekend to ensure everything was okey-dokey. It might even have saved the patient's life.

Mr. Martinez was admitted on a day that proved to be exactly the wrong one in terms of his getting care. I guess the cards just came up wrong for the poor guy. If he'd gotten sick on Wednesday or Friday, he'd probably still be alive today. As it was, he got sick on the one day that would leave him most vulnerable. He was admitted by a team that was taking the last on-call of their current rotation on a Thursday.

A "rotation" is a given amount of time, usually one or two months, that a house officer spends on a particular ward. He may, for example, spend a month doing internal medicine on Cloud, move on to two months in the ICU at NYG, return to the CCU at MH, and so on. In terms of hospital safety nets, the few days that follow each rotation change are the times that the patients, still unfamiliar to their freshly rotated doctors, are most vulnerable. In the case of Mr. Martinez, the hospital safety net was full of holes.

The patient was sent upstairs from the ER at about eleven or twelve at night, looked at once by the resident and once by the intern, and written some brief admitting orders. He was not seen again by a doctor for the rest of the night.

The day following a night on call is traditionally devoted to "mopping up." All stable patients are tucked into bed, and elective procedures and tests are put off until the following day. The intern makes it his business to clean up paperwork, write a short note on each of the patients, and get the hell out of the hospital.

For the team that admitted Mr. Martinez, this particular Friday was not only a ragged, postcall, mop-up, get-the-hell-out-of-the-hospital day, but also the last day of the rotation, a double incentive for a frenzied rush to the exit. The coming weekend might be the first they had completely to themselves for months. They were in so much of a rush, in fact, that on Friday Mr. Martinez, the dirtball junkie, was not seen at all. They were simply too fried to stick around long enough to have a good look at him. They may even have been so fried that they completely forgot the patient was in the hospital.

At MH there'd been an attempt to narrow the holes in the safety net by staggering the rotation change dates of the interns and residents. When a new team of interns arrived the old resident would stay for a few days to familiarize them with their patients. They, in turn, would fill in the new resident when he arrived a day or two later. Rotation change dates were periods that left patients particularly vulnerable, and this plan was meant to ensure that there would be at least one person who'd known the patients for at least a few days.

Mr. Martinez fell onto the safety net and went right through a gigantic hole. The fresh interns arrived on Saturday to "pick up a new service," to assume care of the patients the old interns had left behind. Though the old resident was familiar with the patients and could smooth this task for them, all anyone was really interested in doing on Saturday was, once again, getting out of the hospital. Technically, all they had to do was check out the patients, make sure everyone was alive, and bolt. Under normal circumstances, given long-standing familiarity with the patients on the part of both the interns and resident, this informal policy might have borderline acceptability. The interns could focus on those of their patients they knew to be sickest, work quickly, and not worry about a detailed look at the rest.

The resident, now on his last day on service, arrived early, checked each of the patients with the new interns, and left shortly afterward. The interns, lacking familiarity with each of the patients, simply focused on those they had been told were sickest, leaving the more detailed reviews for Monday. On Saturday, Mr. Martinez, still feverish and vomiting, was seen only briefly.

On Sunday the doctors stayed home.

On Monday the interns, now supposedly familiar with all of their patients, had a new resident. Theoretically, the new resident would spend the day reviewing the patients' charts and examining them. Unfortunately, the team was now once again on call. The day and night were extremely busy. Mr. Martinez was not seen at all.

On Tuesday, the interns and their resident spent the day mopping up after their night on call. Mr. Martinez was not seen until that night, five full days after he'd been admitted, when he died of dehydration and electrolyte abnormalities. His blood chemistry numbers suggested that he'd spent five days crawling around the Sahara rather than as a patient at Manhattan Hospital.

The story of Mr. Martinez illustrates clearly that uncaring and neglect can be very dangerous. It also demonstrates that one reason for such uncaring and neglect is the fact that interns work ridiculous hours, that they simply burn out, and focus on "getting the hell out of the hospital." Nonetheless, there are other, more complex causes behind such behavior, forces that are built right into the system of medical education.

The truth is that most people start the whole miserable business with the right motivations. I've met only one person who came right out and admitted that money was the reason he wanted to go into medicine. He said, "I want to be a doctor because I want lots and lots of money." Poor bastard. If he'd gone into the stock market back in '79 or '80 he'd probably be retired by now. Everyone else I've talked to, even those who were the scummiest to be egested from the system of medical training, started the whole escapade with some sense of wanting to help people, of wanting to contribute in some way. Somewhere along the way a lot of these people were transformed into shitheads, and it really isn't necessary to look very far to find out why.

First of all, as I described earlier, the first lesson learned is that altruism has little to do with success in academia and medicine; what counts is the ability to claw one's way ahead of the competition. In fact, altruism stands in direct opposition to success. A premed who offers help to a struggling fellow premed risks his own chances of getting into medical school. A hot-stuff medical student keeps his mouth shut when a colleague is unable to answer a question posed by the team attending. The lesson learned is: Keep your nose brown, collect brownie points, and look the other way when you observe a colleague making a mistake. Society, speaking out of one side of its mouth, exclaims, "Do unto others as you would have them do unto you." Reality dictates otherwise.

By the time the student arrives at the onset of internship, he has already been preselected to be best not at giving, but at taking, and any fossilized motives to be altruistic lie buried in his experiences in college and med school. This individual, once so bright-eyed, bushy-tailed, and eager to make a contribution to his fellow man, now enters the hospital and is worked into the ground. The new intern is thrown head over heels onto the wards and worked 80 to 120 hours a week into a blubbering pulp, surrounded by shit, illness, death, the noxious, pungent scent of disinfectant, and a stupefying array of the most twisted and egocentric personalities he will ever encounter.

The once stellar achiever, at the top of his class in college and admired for his status as "medical student," is ignominiously shoved to the bottom of the stack. Confronted by senior docs whose egos have been completely destroyed, the intern is told that everything he is doing is totally wrong, the handiwork of a complete asshole. He will be berated by virtually everyone in the hospital, from the chiefs of departments who insist on knowing why such a moron thinks he has the right to call himself "doctor," to lab techs who, believing all doctors are morons by definition, realize that only interns are sufficiently powerless to be informed of this fact.

The intern's salary, broken down to a per hour basis, is under minimum wage. He is at the bottom of the totem pole, the know-nothing, the order taker, the workhorse, the scum sucker. It comes as little surprise that bitterness and uncaring develop, that the prime concern of the average house officer changes from "I want to help people" to "Let's get the hell out of the hospital."

By his superiors, the big-cheese, hot-shot docs, those who are responsible for the shaping of the intern into a real doc, the intern is told, "You're a doctor now, boy! These patients are your damn responsibility! If you don't keep your nose to the grindstone until it's a bloody mess you're going to kill 'em, boy, and it'll be your damn fault! Better stay up till you're ready to drop and then some 'cause if you don't, well, you're just a *bad doc,* boy! Now don't give me any back talk or guff about this, boy, because I've got to go home now, the wife's got dinner on the table. See you in the morning, boy! I expect you'll have looked under the microscope at all the snot on all your patients by then. Well, damn, if you haven't, well you know what that means about what kind of doctor you are! A *bad doctor!* Keep up the good work, boy, and I'll see your sorry ass in the morning!"

The system of medical education is, in fact, totally flawed. It gives students the wrong motivations in college, establishes the wrong criteria to select people for medical school, emphasizes the wrong ways to approach the needs of patients, and just plain abuses interns and residents. What it should be doing is teaching people how to pursue their goal of helping others in a comprehensive manner, both technically and socially. To the housestaff it should say, "We know you want to do good, and we know you're doing your best, and we're going to try to make it as tolerable as possible, and, as unfortunate as it is, we understand that you're going to slip on occasion, but we'll still be on your side." If every student, intern, and resident was told this just once I sincerely believe that doctors in the United States would be a better crowd than they are today.

The cast of characters that results, the kinds of bad docs that get dumped out of the other end of the system, the remnants of the caring human beings who entered college and medical school ten to fifteen years earlier, is scary, fas-

171

cinating, and not all that surprising. Sliding from the top of the heap in college and medical school into a pile of shit, the abuse and paying of dues of internship and residency, can grotesquely inflate and derange the ego of the doc when residency is finally over. The stereotype of the stuck-up, domineering, and egocentric doc is, unfortunately, quite accurate. It seems pristinely clear that after years of having one's face ground into the dirt, one might in turn seek to do some grinding of others' faces, to preen and strut and declare one's invincibility like a rutting goat.

One of my favorite rituals of rutting-goat docs was that of academic one-upmanship. It was taken as a sign of medical virility, especially on ward rounds, to be able to quote in the most seemingly relaxed way the absolute most recent research data about a given medical condition. Residents, senior docs, and hot interns engaged themselves in an orgy of chin rubbing and harrumphing, reciting the details of data to be "released in next week's *New England Journal of Medicine.*"

On one particular evening I had the displeasure of being trapped on rounds in the NYG intensive care unit with Dr. Big, the all-powerful head of the hospital, and Dr. Young and Smart attending, a newly minted private doc who made up for his relative lack of years by being as aggressive and seemingly knowledgeable as possible. If there were two people in the hospital not to get into a one-upmanship scene with, it was Drs. Big and Young and Smart.

Rounds had started with Dr. Big directing the usual barbed accusations of mental retardation and the like at random members of the housestaff, while Dr. Young and Smart stood looking bored, smirking occasionally at Dr. Big's comments. Eventually, to the relief of the housestaff, the senior docs began to pick at each other, and by the time we reached the Man with Hypothermia (or, the Man Who Was Very Cold), their initial sullen parrying had escalated to direct accusations of misinformation.

Apparently, the topic of hypothermia was one that had not been well investigated, and the recommendations regarding treatment had not been agreed upon. It seemed that there was a paucity of data to use for one-upmanship. Dr. Young and Smart believed that the pulseless hypothermic patient was best treated with external cardiac massage until a foul odor indicated the onset of "biologic" death, and Dr. Big believed that treatment more appropriately consisted of electric stimulation of the patient's heart, presumably until the patient was too hot to touch.

The doctors glared at each other, groping wordlessly for the data that would prove themselves right, when Dr. Big suddenly blurted, "The Dachau data clearly indicated that the heart's rhythm degenerates into asystole."

I dropped my clipboard.

Dr. Young and Smart assumed an expression of momentary distaste, and then replied, "Dr. Big, the Dachau data was very poorly controlled; however, as I remember, it indicated ventricular fibrillation as the final rhythm."

The results of Nazi experimentation on living human beings were parried back and forth for a few more sentences until the discussion drifted, as conversations will, onto another subject. No one pointed out to the docs that the use of such "data" in the name of proving oneself academically superior elevated the practice of one-upmanship from the neurotic to the truly inappropriate. These doctors apparently were so insecure that they thought it appropriate to quote the results of Gestapo experimentation at Dachau, in which living human beings were submerged naked in ice water, to prove their own worth.

The training process is so brutal that the behavior of

docs can graduate from borderline to genuine psychosis.

Surgeons, for example, go through a paramilitary residency program that lasts five years, with work hours ranging from the routine weekly minimum of 80 to 120 to literally living in the hospital for weeks at a time. That should be enough to crack just about anyone. The really high-powered blades, like pediatric heart surgeons, train for ten or more years after medical school, and must virtually devote their entire lives to the profession.

The hierarchy among surgeons is firmly established. The foot soldier, or "grunt," is the intern; the sergeant is the second-year resident; the lieutenant a senior resident; the captain, the chief resident; the general, a fifth-year; and the commander in chief, resplendent in silk suit and tie, the attending. As in the military, "shit rolls downhill" in this hierarchy, and the physical and psychological abuse of residents and interns runs rampant.

The following, which occurred to a group of surgical residents at NYG during the last hospital workers' strike, is a perfect example of the kind of mind-boggling mental stresses that docs in training may be forced to endure.

The strike, which involved nonmedical staff, created drastic reductions in housekeeping, maintenance, dietary, lab, and clerical services, which were being provided at minimal levels by nonunion personnel. In order to reduce the strain on these services, the housestaff had been instructed to order routine lab tests only when they were absolutely necessary.

In keeping with this edict, the chief of surgery decided that urine analysis (urinalysis), normally a standard preoperative test, was nonessential and would not be ordered routinely until the strike was over. When absolutely necessary, it would be done by the residents themselves. Naturally, he did nothing to ease the increased work load created by the strike; to the contrary, the pace of the operating schedule actually increased. The housestaff, now

174

more overworked than ever, simply disregarded his directive and continued to order all routine labs as usual.

When he learned that his orders were being disobeyed, the department head blew his top and called a surprise meeting of the senior surgical housestaff to teach his underlings a lesson. The perplexed residents assembled in his office and were directed to five paper cups sitting on his desk. The cups, they were told, contained urine. Reminding the staff never again to forget to follow their orders to the letter, the chief directed the doctors to drink the urine.

Being the big-cheese doc, the head of the department could make or break anyone's career. All the years of abuse and paying of dues would amount to nothing were the residents to stand up to this fantastic antic. So, no one said anything. One or two of them, attempting to defuse the situation, simply laughed and sipped at the containers before them. These actions apparently satisfied the chief enough that he relieved the rest of the same task. He lectured the stunned group on the need to follow orders and then dismissed everyone. It was not clear whether the containers actually held urine.

I was furious when I heard this story, furious that one man had the power to treat people so shabbily and furious that no one in the room stood in the defense of himself or of his coworkers. It would have been so justified for one of the docs to have quietly walked to the front of the room, swept the containers onto the floor, and called an end to such a travesty. Nonetheless, no one did that, and given the situation and the fear engendered by the training process, I understand why.

In light of events like this it's not surprising that people's brains and self-esteem can get seriously scrambled and deranged. The carnage caused by normal human error, neglect, and indifference may be fearsome, but that inflicted by the psychologically twisted is truly the most dangerous and chilling.

A story I like to tell that illustrates this describes the management of a patient with a gunshot wound who was brought into NYG one night.

Reportedly, the patient committed some kind of heinous crime, something on the order of rape or armed robbery. Adding insult to injury, he then got into a shoot-out with the police, and earned himself a brand new shiny red bullet wound to his chest. Once the smoke cleared the cops graciously threw him into a squad car and hauled him into NYG.

On arriving in the ER the man had a bullet hole in his sternum (breast bone) and no blood pressure or pulse. He was brought directly to the rear of the ER, which was set up for surgical emergencies, and set upon by the surgical team on call. Within seconds he was intubated, plugged full of IVs, and administered CPR.

CPR (cardiopulmonary resuscitation) is administered to the pulseless patient in an attempt to restore the circulation of blood. When someone drops dead of a cardiac arrest (complete cessation of the heart) this works fairly well; the pressure of the chest compressions squeezes the heart, mimicking its pumping action. In someone with a bullet hole in his heart, chest compressions serve only to squeeze blood out of the hole rather than into the normal blood vessels to the body. Such was the case with this patient. When the staff checked him for pulses to determine the effectiveness of CPR, they found none, confirming that he had a hole either in his heart or in a nearby large blood vessel.

The surgeons next decided to "crack" (open) the patient's chest. In order to keep his blood inside his blood vessels they would have to open him up and sew closed the hole in his heart. At the same time they would pour fluid and donated blood from the blood bank into the rapist gunman through intravenous lines and, having repaired the hole in the heart, massage it internally (that is, a surgeon would squeeze the heart manually with his hand inside the patient's chest) to keep the blood flowing.

Having done this it might then be possible to restart the heart electronically by shocking, or "defibrillating," it. In a person who hadn't been dead too long or lost too much blood this might result in saving the patient. Admittedly, the odds are fairly bad. There was a long article in *The Village Voice* a few years ago about a guy who got stabbed in the chest right outside the entry to an emergency room of a downtown hospital and managed to survive a scenario like this. I've been involved in similar scenes a good dozen times and have yet to see someone come close to surviving.

Commanding the scene in the ER was the fifth-year surgical resident. Fifth-years spend an extraordinary amount of time in the hospital, months at a time, and are supposed to do nothing but operate and tell the rest of the team what to do for the pre- and postop patients. At night they stay in their on-call rooms and don't leave unless there's a major emergency case in the ER. Living in the hospital and doing nothing but operating is meant as a perk for all the dues paid in reaching the final year.

The scenario orchestrated by the fifth-year was a frenetic and bloody one, with a dozen people crowded around the patient; sundry members of the surgical housestaff, lots of nurses, an overexcited medical student or two, and even an internist peering in from the rear somewhere. Draped ignominiously on a stretcher, soaking in a pool of his own blood, lay the perpetrator himself, his chest held wide open by a big stainless-steel rib retractor while a surgeon fiddled about with his heart.

In a scene like this, blood and garbage is everywhere, blood from the patient and garbage from the equipment used on him: EKG paper, sterile wrappings, used needles and syringes. The doctors are covered with blood. It is on their shoes, pants, shirts, jackets, hands, arms, and spattered on their faces. Three or four years, and hundreds of liters of blood later, many of them will lie awake at night, terrified of having contracted the AIDS virus in any of dozens of identical scenes.

The surgeons crowded around the patient were busy, busy, busy. One was attempting to sew closed the bullet hole in the patient's heart. Another stood at his neck, stabbing him over and over to place a central line. There was probably even one at his thigh attempting a slash femoral cutdown, the most macho way to put in an IV. Once, while participating in a similar scene, I asked the chief if he wanted me to place a line. Without answering he glanced down and slashed open (thus the name) a four-inch wound on the front of the patient's thigh. I grasped the upper and lower edges of the wound and gave a good strong tug, pulling back skin and fat to reveal the saphenous vein. I lifted the vein with a hemostat, made a small slit on one side, and poked an IV right into it. The whole procedure was exceedingly emphatic and gratifying.

That the current patient had been dead for fifteen minutes or a half hour, and had possibly been taken on a quick tour of the neighborhood by the cops before his arrival in the ER, was not lost on the surgical team. His failure to fall into the category of innocent bystander would also influence the extent and quality of the care he received.

Having put on a grand spectacle of slashing and sewing, transfusing a unit or two of blood, and zapping the patient's long-dead heart with a few blasts from the defibrillator paddles, the fifth-year decided to end the show, dispatch the staff to their other duties, and light up a cigarette. He pulled the curtain around the stretcher and leaned against the wall.

He glanced at the second-year, who was sewing the gaping chest wound closed with coarse, wide-set sutures before

178

sending the body to the morgue. "So, what's the deal? Why'd the cops shoot this guy?"

The second-year didn't look up. "Well, they said that there was a rape, or something like that, and, uh, then there was a shoot-out, and I guess the cops shot the guy."

The fifth-year nodded, walked over to the patient, right up next to the still-open surgical wound, took the cigarette out of his mouth, and flicked it into the patient's chest cavity.

He looked up at his colleague. "Yeah? Well, fuck him." He then walked out of the ER and returned to his on-call room.

There was another interesting case, a woman who'd been involved in a domestic dispute involving a loaded shotgun. She came into the NYG ER one night when I wasn't there, but I was told that someone had put a shotgun a foot in front of her face and blown half of it neat and clean, right off. She walked into the emergency room breathing and talking just like a regular person except that she was missing a big piece of her head.

The reason the story is interesting (bad injuries being nothing new to most medical stories) is that the surgeons went completely bananas, running around taking Polaroid pictures of the woman and her face and just about everything else in a kind of a surgical feeding frenzy. Everybody was pretty amazed and interested by the patient herself until the surgeons started making such a spectacle of themselves, and then everyone began watching them instead.

I know the essential parts of this story to be true because a few days later one of my surgical friends shoved several wallet-sized close-up snaps of the woman under my nose.

I said, "Christ, what happened to her?" and he told me the medical details. Later, one of the nurses told me the rest of the story. I don't know what eventually happened to the woman, though I heard she survived.

You really couldn't blame the surgeons for getting into their work the way they did, for their uncanny ability to dissociate operating from the people they were operating on. It was just their way of adjusting to having the stuff crammed in their faces twenty-four hours a day, seven days a week, for five long years.

In discussing iatrogenic causes of illness, I've covered problems ranging from the odd, well-intentioned (though lethal) mistake, to the actions of the truly deranged.

It would be greatly remiss of me to omit the problem of substance abuse among doctors. Doctors have among the highest rates of drug abuse, alcoholism, divorce, depression, suicide, and sundry other forms of social pathology of any professional group. Within the profession those who are drunks or junkies are cryptically referred to as "impaired physicians."

The extent of substance-abuse-induced iatrogenic injury is staggering. When I was in training I was just one doctor in one hospital and I heard many stories about docs who were either drinking too much or dabbling much too heavily in controlled substances, including surgeons who went to work stoned. One got high before going to work in the emergency room to "mellow out," as though working there were akin to having a stroll in the park. Another racked up his car three times. My experience is not anecdotal, and everyone in the health care field has similar horror stories.

10

The Caring Doc

The truth of the matter was that, at least as a resident or intern, it wasn't possible to be the ideal physician, the caring, feeling, dedicated-to-the-pit-of-the-soul doctor, the kind of doctor that I've described as being a "good doc." Anybody who did this would go crazy, plain and simple. How would it be possible to be so caring and heartfelt about a miasma of illness, most of which one could do little or nothing about? How could it be possible, especially at the training level, when it seemed that everyone was going out of their way to grind the intern's face in the dirt, and then complain about the bloodstains left on their shoes? The answer is that it wasn't possible. It was sane to not care. Later, when life became a little more normal, when one's hours became those of the almighty senior docs, those of us who survived with our egos intact, those of us who hadn't been transformed into the next generation of egomaniacs, could rebuild our sense of caring and compassion. Residency was a time to build barriers for protection of the soul, and to hope that later, years down the road, the barriers might slowly come back down again.

The reality was that it wasn't important to be a caring doc. It wasn't important to give even the slightest drab of a shit about anyone. What was important was to *behave* like a caring doc, to take excellent care of the patients *as though* you really did give a shit, even if you didn't.

When I was an intern, I remembered a time four impossibly long years before, when I'd entered medical school all bright-eyed and bushy-tailed and believed right in the pit of my much younger soul that yes, by God, I was going into all of this because I did indeed want to help people. I miraculously survived the cutthroat competition of college, cruising along and getting good grades as though I were being guided by a guardian angel. My liberal, eggheaded parents supported me every step of the way, all the time nurturing the sentiment that my motivations were good ones, that in the end I'd be well prepared to help my fellow man. I came out of college with little hate, still eager to be of use to people. I remembered these sentiments when I was an intern, but it was as though I was remembering the motivations of a character in a book I'd read sometime in the past. Somewhere in my past there was another person with my name and body who gave such a high-and-mighty damn about people.

When I was an intern that person wasn't dead, but certainly in a deep sleep. As an intern I floated along amidst shit and death, decent and kind people devastated by horrendous illness, and listened to my seniors, my role models, discussing the research efforts of the Gestapo. As an intern, I fixated on one single idea: "Get me the hell out of this place before I crack completely."

To tell the truth, I wasn't even sure that the nauseatingly bright-eyed, eager-beaver do-gooder within me was only asleep. He was so much of a foreign concept that I couldn't tell if maybe he really was dead, never to wake up again. I did know, though, that all along I'd been brought up to believe that I was supposed to do good. Society said, "Do good!" Graduation speeches said, "Do good!" Fine literature said, "Do good!" My family and upbringing said, "Do good!" I understood the idea, I knew that the most accepted and respected of individuals were the ones who "did good!" I knew this, but as an intern I really didn't feel it; the idea of doing good for its own sake had no appeal at all.

I suppose that in the end I *behaved* like someone who cared, I went through the *motions* of someone who did good, I did what I understood to be the *right thing* for all my patients because I knew that not doing so would turn me from a "caring doc" into a "bad doc." Maybe I *did good* because I feared failing the teachings of my upbringing, and becoming the kind of doc that society, in its two-faced way, frowned upon. Maybe the dead bright-eyed guy would one day wake up, and I'd be glad I'd done good because once again it would be important to me for its own sake.

Nonetheless, let me assure you that as an intern, I really didn't care. I didn't care, for example, about the Lady with Lung Cancer.

I admitted the Lady with Lung Cancer to the ICU one day about six months into my internship, a period when I was especially depressed, when the months of internship already past felt like years, and those ahead felt like decades.

The Lady with Lung Cancer was a patient of Dr. Cancer, poor, dead Mr. Smith's private doc. Like Mr. Smith, she had been treated with a grisly assortment of toxic medications, drugs that were designed to "kill all rapidly dividing cells!" Likewise, she suffered their toxic side effects, especially the "bottoming out" of her white blood cells, her body's defense against infection. Unlike Mr. Smith, she had been treated as an outpatient rather than in the hospital. She went to get injected with the drugs at Doc Cancer's office once every few weeks.

183

About two days before her arrival, near dead, in the hospital, the patient had discovered a few funny-looking blisters on her arm. Within twenty-four hours the blisters had spread over her whole body. On the day of admission she'd collapsed at home and was taken to the hospital where she was found to be in shock, trying very hard to die.

In medicine, "shock" refers to a catastrophic drop in blood pressure, and has no connection to its popular meaning, a stuporous psychologic response to a traumatic event, a state of stunned surprise. There are several different kinds of medical shock: cardiogenic shock (low blood pressure resulting from a failing heart), burn shock, traumatic shock (for example, a patient develops low blood pressure while bleeding to death from a gunshot wound), and septic shock, to name a few. All of them have the same result: dangerously low blood pressure.

Septic shock is caused by overwhelming infection, like that occurring when a cancer patient gets his bone marrow atom-bombed and runs out of white blood cells. In septic shock the body is staggered by infection. Millions and billions of little germs, like the infamous Red Chinese hordes of the Korean War, take over the bloodstream and disperse toxins, like Communist propaganda, that cause the blood vessels to dilate and collapse. Good tight blood vessels (this sounds admittedly sexual, the proper medical phrase is "adequate vascular tone") are as necessary to maintain blood pressure as a well-functioning heart. In septic shock "vascular collapse" is the chief cause of shock.

The Lady with Lung Cancer was brought to the ICU where I stuck her with a great big central line and poured in bottles and bottles of saline to help bring up her blood pressure. This didn't work very well, probably because all of her blood vessels were collapsed, so I started her on a "vasoactive" drug called dopamine, a medication designed to narrow the arteries and make her heart beat faster and harder, two actions that would elevate her blood pressure. This combination of fluids and pressors, as saline and dopamine are called, started to work, and her blood pressure rose from 50 to 80, about two thirds normal.

I'd been working on the patient for an hour or two when Dr. Cancer wandered by to see how she was doing. He was particularly concerned about her white blood cell count, and asked me if her complete blood count (or CBC) had come back from the hematology lab. A CBC details everything anyone could ever want to know about a patient's red and white blood cells (as well as their platelets, which help blood clot): how many there are, what they look like, etc.

I handed him the slip, which was fresh from the lab. A normal white count ranges from 5,000 to 8,000. The patient's was under 100. Dr. Cancer looked at the slip, looked up at me, and then looked at the floor without speaking. This was the oncologist's nightmare; blasting a patient with chemo in the hope of shrinking the tumor, and winding up dropping his white count and puttting him into septic shock.

"I killed her."

I mustered up an expression of seriousness. "Listen, the lady has lung cancer, all you were doing was treating her. I patted him on the shoulder and returned to work.

Having precariously stabilized the patient, who lay unconscious in a bed, I was now obligated to carry out the ceremonial torture work-up, testing designed to determine where exactly she was infected, and what bacteria had caused her to go into septic shock. I might add that the rotation I was working in the ICU was two weeks, twenty-four on/twenty-four off, a schedule that no self-respecting union would allow for its members, and is only pulled off by doctors and soldiers. Being now on the last day of the rotation and twelve hours into the shift, I commenced the work-up of the patient without the itty-bittiest

185

trace, not an inkling, not a drab of a sense of caring. I did what I had to do because for whatever reason—be it fear of being a social outcast, worrying that sometime later I would become a born-again do-gooder, concern that I'd get sued if I just sat down and let the patient box—I understood that at a minimum I had to *behave* like a do-gooder doctor, like a doctor who cared.

Nothing would have made me happier than for someone to have come in and said, "Go home, I'll spend the next twelve hours torturing this woman, leave it to me. Go home and rest." I believe I'd even have been satisfied with, "Guess what?! Morality has been officially changed! Now, the idea is to *kill* patients instead of *cure* them! So, now you can just leave her to God's will, and *go home!*"

No one came in and made either remark so I commenced the good-doctor routine. I cleaned four different spots on the patient's arms and drew four sets of blood cultures. I helped the nurse stick a catheter up the lady's urethra into her bladder and sent off a specimen of pee for culture. I stuck a thin catheter down her nose, sucked some snot up out of her lungs, and sent that off for culture, too. Because she was unconscious, the patient offered no resistance to any of this, as had Uncle Melvin, my old, demented sumo wrestler patient on Cloud. In fact, that she was unconscious made all of my tasks much easier. I called the X-ray technician and asked him to bring his moaning, beeping, elephantine, dinosaurlike portable X-ray machine and take a picture of her lungs. Because she wasn't breathing too well I intubated her, and hooked her up to a respirator. I stuck in an A-line, a catheter that goes into the radial artery in the wrist and stays there, and attached it to a machine that would display the patient's blood pressure, both digitally and graphically, twenty-four hours a day.

I believed A-lines to be very handy. In addition to providing a constant readout of blood pressure, obviating the fuss with old-fashioned blood pressure cuffs, an A-line could, by virtue of a little stopcock, be used to drain off a dollop of blood without having to stick the patient. As an intern, I believed that every patient in the hospital should have an A-line. By connecting it to a port in the wall, one might theoretically shoot dollops of blood effortlessly to any lab in the hospital with a push of a button. Whenever a blood test was needed, rather than using old-fashioned syringes, needles, alcohol wipes, test tubes, and the rest of it, the intern would simply hit a button on a bedside panel. A little sample of blood would be sucked from the A-line and zipped off to the laboratory just like the sucking pneumatic tube system used to rocket bits of paper through the bowels of the hospital. It would be the intern's ideal labor-saving device.

The only problem I could envision was the possibility of a button getting stuck without the intern or patient realizing it, say, while the patient was asleep. By dollops, the patient would be slowly sucked of blood until dead. Then again, who'd be to blame?

Having collected copious blood, urine, and snot, I rolled the lady over on her side, flexed her legs at the hips and knees, and set about the lumbar puncture, or LP. Known popularly as a "spinal tap," the LP would tell me whether all the little hordes of bugs had entered the patient's nervous system and spine. After a ten-second debate with myself on the need for local anesthesia in the comatose patient, I elected to give her the benefit of the doubt, a behavior I believed emulated that of the now totally mysterious "caring doctor," and squirted a few cc of local anesthetic into the area of her back where I would stick the spinal needle.

Gloved and sterile, I pushed the fine five-inch-long needle between two vertebrae at the base of the spine, aiming it slightly upward, toward the patient's head. After a few inches the needle struck something hard, meaning that instead of guiding the needle between vertebrae, I had bumped into the bone itself. I pulled the needle back, redirected, and again pushed. Again it struck bone. I must have stuck the patient six or seven times, each time coming up against bone. Mumbling that the patient must have bone spurs, or an altered spinal anatomy preventing entry into the canal, I asked the Indian anesthesiologist to give it a try.

He walked over and poked the needle right in, saying, "No problem. No problem."

I collected four quarter-full tubes of bright clear spinal fluid, the watery liquid that bathes the brain and central nervous system, and sent them off for various tests.

The caring, complete, thorough doc would now examine each of the patient's body fluids — pus, snot, urine, and cerebrospinal fluid — under the microscope to determine which of her organ systems were infected. Cursing out loud, I carried the specimens to the lab, layered a sample of each on a slide, and stained them with blue and red dye that would make bacteria stand out. The dye dribbled off the slides, staining my hands red and blue as well as the bugs. In fact, because of the frequency with which I was staining people's body fluids for examination under the microscope, I spent the entire internship year with red-and-blue-stained hands.

The Lady with Lung Cancer had septic shock because she was a cancer patient with a desperate shortage of white blood cells, the perfect setup for a rampant infection. I examined the fluid from the funny-looking pimples first. They were the most likely source of the infestation. Peering into an area smaller than a pinpoint, I saw jillions of little, tiny oval blue critters, none other than staphylococci (or "staph"), the bugs the Aussie doc had discussed on public television. Staph are the kinds of germs docs refer to as "extremely virulent," and when a person gets blood-borne infections with them, he's in a heap of trouble. Only the pus revealed them; that they had spread from the weird pimples all over the patient's body into her bloodstream would be confirmed later, when the bacteriology lab called to announce that "four out of four of the blood cultures were positive for gram positive cocci in clusters."

I sat at the nurses' station. A nearby group of nurses were engaged in reading and answering Trivial Pursuit questions, an activity that seemed to have been going on for several hours. I took the patient's chart down from the chart rack and wrote the history and physical exam, all the available lab values, what I had seen under the microscope, my assessment of what was wrong, and the options for treatment. I did not include the most important and final question to be answered for patients such as this: "Oak or pine?"

Dr. Cancer was still hanging around, seemingly in need of further lamentations about his patient.

"The Lady with Cancer," he began, "is about to become a grandmother for the first time. Both she and her daughter wanted her to stay alive at least until the baby was born."

I asked, "When's the baby due?"

He replied, "About two months. I was trying to give her two more months."

I nodded and returned to writing in the chart. Dr. Cancer sighed heavily and walked out of the ICU.

I finished the note and went outside to talk to the patient's family. They were waiting in the small, stale, cigarette-smoke-scented family waiting area a few steps from the entrance to the ICU. I straightened my tie and ran my hands through my hair. The outward demeanor I projected while working, "I'm stuck in this place torturing dead people for another twelve hours," was not intended for public consumption. For the family, I would straighten my back and shoulders, remove my hands from my pockets, change "yeah" and "nah" to "yes" and "no," and bend myself into my "caring doctor" best. It was an image that said, "I'm doing everything I can for your relative and will keep you informed. You can count on me."

I boldly entered the "family waiting area" and approached the relatives: a sister, a pregnant daughter, and a sympathetic son-in-law. The daughter delivered the standard concerned, straightforward introductory statement.

"I'm the Lady with Lung Cancer's daughter, Mrs. Pregnant with First Grandchild. You must be Dr. Intern. Dr. Cancer told us you'd be taking care of my mother while she is here."

"Yes. Pleased to meet you." I shook her hand.

"How is my mother doing?" The daughter's eyes translated her words. They said, "Lay it on the line, no beating around the bush."

I held her gaze. "Well, to be very candid with you, she is critically ill at the present, though by using fluids and medications we've managed to stabilize her." Translated: "She is sick as shit and will probably die tomorrow."

"What exactly is the problem?"

"We're going on a working diagnosis of septic shock. As you know, the cancer treatment carries the risk of infection. It appears that your mother has been overwhelmed by a small infection that spread rapidly and entered the bloodstream where it caused her blood pressure to drop." People seemed to be reassured by technical jargon, even if they didn't understand its meaning. They assumed it meant their relative was getting the most advanced care possible.

"Unfortunately, right now she is critically ill."

Translated: "Your mother is sick as shit and will probably die tomorrow."

The daughter pushed on. "What will you be able to do for her?"

"Well, we've done everything we can to determine exactly what kind of infection she has and now we've started her on antibiotics, fluids by vein, and drugs to help keep her blood pressure up." Translated: "There's no 'we,' there's just me, a still-pimply kid six months out of medical school, and I've gone through the same routine I do for everyone who is sick as shit and will probably die tomorrow."

"Do you think she will have a chance to see her grandchild? All we wanted to do was have her live until the baby was born." The tone loosens as the daughter begins to cry. She knows how to translate what I've told her.

"There is no way I can tell you whether she will live, only God knows that." I am by no means religious or even a believer in God. Nonetheless, God is useful in situations like this to shift responsibility, and sometimes seems to comfort people.

"I can tell you that without treatment she will certainly pass away [when speaking with relatives permitted words to be used in place of "kick," "tube," "box," "head for Cloud Nine," "go to the eternal care unit," "buy it," "code," and "team" are "pass away" and "expire"; never say "die"], and that treatment offers a chance she will see her grandchild." Translated: "Untreated she'll definitely die, treated she'll probably die," i.e., the Great Medical Hedge.

"Thank you, Doctor. May we go in and see her now?"

"Let me have a few more minutes with her and then I'll come back out to let you in." Translated: "She's unconscious, lying naked and spotted with blood on the bed, and the sheets are on the floor. Her legs are wide open with a catheter trailing out of her crotch and there are syringe wrappers, used needles, and other bits of garbage lying all over the bed, and it'll take me a few minutes to clean up these signs of the cold-bloodedness with which we have welcomed her into Manhattan Hospital."

"All right. Thank you again."

191

That shift marked my last in the ICU and I remember that the patient did make it through the night.

My feelings as an intern went far beyond a lost sense of compassion. Internship was damn hard and I vomited up some much harsher feelings, feelings that did not make me proud. Today, I try to be philosophic about them: "Well, those were some valuable insights that I had into my psyche," and crap like that. At the time they were very painful.

For me, the early morning hours of a night on call were the hardest. Having worked myself to a state of exhaustion, the day-to-day facade, the desire to "do good," to "contribute to my fellow man," wore down, uncovering the more fundamental, raw components of my psyche. And, when the going got tough, these aspects of my "self" emerged in full bloom.

For the people at MH who were up all night on call, the responsibility to admit new patients ended at six-thirty in the morning. Any patient who came onto the ward from the ER after that was a "baby-sit." The on-call intern admitted the patient and wrote orders but, when the rest of the staff arrived in the morning, the patient was transferred to another team. The on-call intern simply "baby-sat" the patient for a few hours.

The period between four-thirty and six-thirty in the morning was the most nerve-wracking of all. Before four-thirty the intern didn't have much reason to believe he wouldn't get any more "hits" (intern's slang for admissions) for the night. After four-thirty, though, he'd get to thinking that if the gods were with him there was a chance the ER would shut up for just two more hours and the only possible admission for the rest of the night would be a baby-sit. Every time his beeper went off for that two-hour period he'd freeze and brace himself to hear the phone number for the ER.

The gods do not side with interns. I was paged for many, many admissions during this time of ulcerogenic suspense, patients who arrived at 6:29 A.M. and were so sick that I wouldn't get a chance to even glance at the rest of my charges until late the following afternoon. It was at these times that the really black, festering feelings came bubbling up, when I'd close my eyes and pray, "Please, God, both you and I know that this character is going to die sometime really soon, right? So what's the big deal if you arrange for a quick power failure and let him die while he's stuck in the elevator coming up from the ER? Huh?"

Sometimes, a patient would elect to get critically ill at the exact instant I was getting on the elevator to leave the hospital. My beeper would scream, "Dr. Intern!! Call blah, blah, blah, blah . . . STAT [fast]! Call blah, blah, blah, blah . . . STAT!"

I'd answer the page at the phone right next to the hospital entrance. "Dr. Intern!" the nurse would shriek, "Mrs. Nearly Dead has a blood pressure of forty and a temp of one-oh-eight!"

Then the thoughts were not quite so restrained. I'd close my eyes tight, pleading vigorously, "Okay, lady, I want you to die right this very minute, so I'm not stuck in this dump from now until doomsday. Be a good patient and die now. Die, die, die, *die!!*" The best admission is no admission, and the next best a dead admission.

I began my work on Cloud as a brand-spanking-new intern in a state of total bewilderment. I was so shocked by the surrealism of the situation for the first few weeks that it didn't occur to me to get angry. Then, late one evening about a month after starting, I found myself wishing death on a poor, hapless, elderly patient who lay floundering before me, sick as a dog, demanding, demanding, demanding care that I had no interest in providing. I stood looking at the patient, listening to her rhythmic moaning, getting angrier and angrier and angrier, and wishing her to die as passionately as I possibly could. Finally, I became so distracted that I was unable to work at all, and went to the nurses' station to sit down and collect myself.

Suddenly, I felt a wave of guilt. How could I have such thoughts, I lamented, how could I actually wish such evil on this poor gork of a patient? What was wrong with me? What happened to all that stuff about being a liberal, about wanting to help people? I returned to the patient feeling guilty and frustrated and forced myself to do what was necessary for her.

I now had a new cause for misery, a charming emotional triple whammy of anger, pain, and remorse. I'd have a truly ugly thought about throwing a patient through the window, and immediately feel guilty for it. For weeks I wondered if the death of my sense of compassion meant I had cracked completely, that I would soon be discovered and committed to a loony bin. Then, quite suddenly and out of the blue, I realized that fantasizing did not constitute a crime. After all, I was being beaten over the head with a daily diet of death, pain, shit, and the constant smell of ammonia. Who wouldn't feel grim? Besides, I wasn't about to actually garrote a patient to avoid providing medical care for him, no matter how crummy I was feeling, or how heartfelt and real the violent sentiment. If Burroughsesque fantasies helped deal with being there, all the better.

This short train of thought came as a major relief, and I soon allowed myself to drift into detailed and violent fantasies without feeling a stitch of guilt. Sometimes I dreamed of my entire patient load dying simultaneously, and of spending the rest of the day watching television. At other times I focused on individual patients. For example, I might be sitting at a patient's bedside at four in the morning, trying to put an IV into intensely small and frail veins. If the patient had any kind of mental status I'd say, "I'm really sorry to wake you, Mr. Small and Frail Veins, but your six A.M. dose of medications is almost due so I have to replace your IV. I'll do my best to get it done quickly." My inner sentiment was markedly different: "If I ever get my hands on the sorry-ass nurse who woke me up for this I'm going to tear her into little teeny, tiny bits of bloody macerated flesh. And then when I'm done with her, Mr. Small and Frail Veins, I'm going to come back in here and stick this IV into your eyeball." Then the IV would pop into a vein and I'd say, "See that? Nothing to it. You can get back to sleep now."

Of course, not everyone adjusted to internship in the same way. Anger and vindictiveness may have been a special, psychotic means of dealing with the hospital unique to myself only. My dedicated compatriot Dolores, for example, was quite different. We were often on call together and, as the night wore on and I became angrier and angrier, she'd descend into the depths of sadness and lament.

Early one morning Dolores was paged to replace someone's IV. I had a note to write in a chart at a nearby nurses' station and accompanied her to the patient's room. She emerged some fifteen minutes later, her head hanging as though she'd just discovered life didn't really have any meaning after all.

I said, "What's the matter?"

She hung her head lower, mumbling, "That poor man."

I said, "Did you get the line in?"

She answered, "No, no. I tried three or four times but I couldn't get the line in. That poor man." Then she sat down at the nurses' station, put her head on the desk, and fell asleep.

I sat looking at her for a minute and decided to try to

put the line in for her. I wouldn't be putting the line in for the patient, I'd be doing it for my friend Dolores. I walked into the patient's room and found a comatose man, intubated and on a respirator, lying in bed all swollen up and soggy like a rotten vegetable. He was swollen from head to foot, a condition called anasarca. I pressed his arm with my thumb. It sank into his flesh and almost disappeared completely. Somewhere inside his gigantic swollen arms were veins into which poor old Dolores was supposed to stick an IV. I took a tourniquet out of my pocket, tied it around his arm, and twiddled my thumbs waiting for a vein to swell up. After a bit I found one I might be able to stick and poked an IV through the patient's skin, which was frail and without turgor. Infinitesimally thin and powdery, it offered no resistance to the needle at all. I managed to get the needle into the vein but it too was very frail and fell apart immediately, bleeding into the surrounding tissue. In intern's lingo, this was called "blowing" the IV.

As soon as I'd walked into the room and seen the patient, I'd accused him in my mind of subjecting my comrade to cruel and unusual punishment just by virtue of being alive. He'd developed anasarca intentionally, to torture interns who would have to put in IVs. After my third try I mentally tossed his bloated body through the unopenable hospital window and watched it make a muffled, juicy splat on the pavement six stories below. After the fourth try I gave up, walked back to the nurses' station, and sat down next to Dolores. She'd awakened from her short nap.

She looked up at me. I said, "I mean who really gives a shit whether or not that guy gets a line or not? He sure as hell doesn't."

Dolores put her head back down on her arms and mumbled into her sleeve, "That poor man."

I folded my arms on the desk in front of me and laid

my head on them. "I mean the best thing for the guy would've been to have died around three weeks ago."

Dolores shifted a little bit and mumbled again, "That poor, poor man."

Then we both fell asleep.

Other people, other friends of mine, had yet other ways of reacting, different ways of coping with the miasma. A guy named Charlie Miller was one of the terrific people I worked with as an intern. Charlie was incredibly young to be a doctor. He'd skipped three years of grade school because he was so smart and then entered a six-year medical program right out of high school, combining college and medical school. As a result Charlie was amazingly young, around twenty-one, while the rest of us were in our mid- to late twenties. Some of the interns had done other things before going to medical school and were in their mid- or late thirties. Charlie was the youngest doctor in the hospital. There were medical students around who were ten years older than he.

One of the wonderful things about Charlie was his blunt and sincere honesty about how much he was mystified by medicine. He was extraordinarily dedicated to the work that baffled him so, and paid little attention to his own needs, walking around the hospital wearing disheveled, blotched whites, with his hair plastered to the thin layer of sweat on his forehead. He had incredibly bright brown eyes that sparkled when he spoke, no matter how long he'd been awake and on his feet. The best time to talk to him was at four in the morning, when everyone was running on automatic and his perplexity was at its peak.

One night Charlie was working in the intensive care unit, and I bumped into him in the hall and asked him how things were going. He was standing in the middle of the hallway holding an X ray up to a fluorescent light, looking at it as though it were a tablet of hieroglyphics.

He looked at me with his sparkling eyes and said, "Well, you know I've got to admit to you that I've got a bunch of patients up there in the ICU and I really don't have any idea of whether they're too wet or too dry or what the heck is going on." Charlie was too nice a guy to use profanity. He was one of those guys without a mean bone in his body.

I said, "Well, why don't you ask your resident? I mean after all there's supposed to be someone around who has at least some idea of what's going on, right?"

Charlie shrugged. "Well, yeah, I know what you mean by that, but to tell you the truth I really haven't seen my resident for the last few hours. I think he went to sleep or something."

My beeper started shrieking about making a phone call "STAT!" I moved to the door to the stairs and looked back at him. "Well, anyhow, good luck, Charlie." I zipped into the stairwell, leaving Charlie standing in the hall, the X ray still suspended in midair below the fluorescent light.

Charlie's luck was so bad the year I was an intern that it became popular to refer to a particularly sick patient as a "Miller admission." Charlie would get people who were sick as dogs when he was on call, almost without fail. One day an old lady he had been taking care of on Cloud kicked the bucket. She was terribly frail and though everybody agreed that she was sick, nobody could figure out exactly what was wrong. Mostly, she sat in bed and complained, "I feel sick," and looked worse and worse and worse, sagging farther and farther and farther over in bed until her chin was almost resting in her lap. Charlie got all the X rays and blood tests his resident and attending could dream up for him to get but never came up with anything that was definitely wrong.

I'd say to him, "So, Charlie, that lady of yours looks

pretty sick, what's her problem?"

He'd look puzzled, like he usually did, and say, "Well, you know, to tell you the truth I really can't seem to figure out just what it is that's bothering her, but, yeah, she does look pretty sick."

I had a patient in the same room and one day I happened to notice Charlie's patient sitting bolt-upright in bed glaring around the room with great big shining eyeballs. I didn't pay much attention to this and about a half hour later a code was called and I jogged into the room to find Charlie bent over her doing chest compressions, as she was now dead.

He looked up at me and said, "You know, we never did quite figure out what was wrong with this lady."

Charlie had been on call the night before and was looking more harried and disheveled than usual. He was covered with the thin, dull layer of sweat characteristic of the day after call. Naturally, he'd been about to wrap up the day's work and head home when the lady tubed.

Charlie's problem wouldn't be in patient care. The patient would be subjected to coding, the humiliation of advanced cardiac life support, for a half hour or forty minutes and then sent on up to Cloud 9, the certainty in ninety-nine out of one hundred codes. The problem would be the paperwork, filling out the notorious death certificate, notifying the family, and so on. These tasks kept the average intern in the hospital at least an hour extra and could potentially tie Charlie down for two or three. It was a perfect moment for generating a black mood.

Charlie wasn't the kind of guy to come out with something like, "The least she could've done, if she was going to die anyhow, was to do it a bit earlier in the day so I'd have a chance to get out of here on time." Instead, he stared down at the patient, who was now covered with blood and garbage from the code, shaking his head. Then he looked up at me, started to say something, stopped, and looked back down again, as though he'd thought better of his comment.

Finally, he looked back up and said, "You know what really gets me? I'll tell you. What really gets me is that today was going to be the first day that I'd be able to get out of here by five P.M. since I started working in this place. That's what gets me. It really does." Those were the cruelest words I ever heard Charlie speak.

I had another friend, a surgeon, who had his own unique way of dealing with the hospital. Though he was technically skilled, he didn't even pretend to care about his patients, and made no bones about it. As far as I was concerned, this meant that he would inevitably become a "bad doc," the kind of surgeon I wouldn't even allow to operate on my dog. Still, we got along, and helped each other through the night when we were on call together, joking and laughing and complaining about being interns.

I was sitting with him at one of the nurses' stations one night when his beeper went off. He'd always swear and complain when he was paged because it meant more work. He wrinkled his face, exclaimed, "Shit!" and dialed the number to find out what task lay in store. He grunted at the receiver. "This is Dr. Surgical Intern! What's the goddam problem?"

There was a pause of a second or two and then his voice became suddenly low and sultry. He said, "Oh. . . ! Hi. . . ! How are you? What's going on?" I raised my eyebrows and looked up from the chart I was writing in.

A few more seconds went by and he said, "Yeah, yeah . . . How about fifteen minutes, Okay?" He paused another second, listening, and then hung up the phone.

I looked at him and smiled broadly. "You bastard! I bet your friggin' wife doesn't know about this, does she?"

He returned my smile with a grin and then sauntered off the ward.

My friend's arrangement was a great one, one that I both envied and resented. He had a friend, or possibly a few friends, a nurse here, a tech or a clerk there, who paged him whenever they had a break to find out if he was free to disappear off into a closet for a quickie. He'd disappear for fifteen minutes or a half hour and come back with a classic shit-eating grin on his face, and all of a sudden it looked like being on call wasn't such a terrible thing for him after all.

11

I Could Only Laugh

The question that remains to be answered, a question I posed some time back, is an obvious one. Why is the system of medical training the way it is? Why are interns and residents worked to the bone for forty hours at a shot, three times a week, five years at a stretch, leaving their egos ragged and sometimes unsalvageable? What is the purpose of all of this bullshit?

As I mentioned earlier, the response of the typical hard-nosed American Medical Association type to this question usually regards the ill-founded belief that it somehow hardens a doc, teaches him how to function under stress, gives him "balls." This, of course, isn't the reason at all. The answer is simple and straightforward. The system is the way it is because of *money*. Take an example.

Mr. Heart Attack is a nice gentleman in his fifties who comes into the hospital one day having a big-time heart attack. In the course of his hospital stay, there will be about fifty people involved in Mr. Heart Attack's care. Following the pecking order: There is his private doctor, Manhattan Hospital's big-cheese heart specialist, Dr. Heart. Then there are Dr. Heart's associates, Dr. Heart Surgeon and Dr. Heart Tests. A few nonheart specialists may become involved in Mr. Heart Attack's care, such as Dr. Neurologist (Dr. Nerves) and Dr. Gastroenterologist

(Dr. Stomach and Intestines). Their skills will be critical if Mr. Heart Attack feels some numbness in his left pinky or has an episode of vomiting.

Consultants tend to multiply in a plaguelike fashion, and Dr. Heart's associates will bring in associates of their own. Dr. Heart Surgeon, for example, specializes in octuple heart bypass operations and works hand in hand with Dr. Vascular Surgeon (Dr. Veins). Should Dr. Heart Surgeon decide to operate on Mr. Heart Attack's heart, a possibility correlating directly with the allure of next year's Jaguar sedan, Doc Veins's skills will prove indispensable. He will chop blood vessels out of the patient's legs, trim them nicely and plug up any holes, and give them to Dr. Heart Surgeon to use in rearranging the flow of traffic in Mr. Heart Attack's heart.

Way below the Drs. Private is Dr. Cardiology Fellow, the guy training to become a big-cheese heart doc. When Mr. Heart Attack is admitted, the Drs. Private speak with Dr. Cardiology Fellow and tell him what they want done with their patient. Next, pecking order-wise, is the resident. The resident consults with Dr. Cardiology Fellow and Dr. Heart, and carefully builds a massive collection of scut for the intern who works in the cardiac care unit (CCU). Next is the CCU nursing staff, men and women who do most of the nitty-gritty of patient care, giving meds, taking vitals, counseling the patient, etc. Next are the Allied Medical Professionals: physical and occupational therapists who will later rehabilitate Mr. Heart Attack, X-ray techs who take his fifty X rays, electrocardiogram techs who take fourteen EKGs a day, dietary workers who bring him bland, salt-free food, custodial people who help clean up after the docs and nurses, blood drawers who drain his body of blood, an army of clerical and bureaucratic personnel who ensure that the hospital gets paid, and chart reviewers who placate the insurance companies by telling them they don't have to pay for the occasional patient. Finally, way, way below, bleary-eyed, trailing around a pocketful of dirty needles and a scut list, wandering up and down the corridors seeking blood tests long ago stuffed into a lab coat pocket, there is the intern.

Mr. Heart Attack spends a few days in the hospital but his heart attack pain doesn't go away. He is taken to see Dr. Heart Tests, who sticks a tube up near his heart arteries, releases dye, and takes very fancy X-ray pictures demonstrating that his heart arteries are hopelessly clogged from a lifetime of cigarette smoking, fatty food, lack of exercise, and plush living. The procedure takes an hour. Dr. Heart glances at the pictures, assumes a very stern expression, and calls Dr. Heart Surgeon on the phone. Dr. Heart Surgeon (who keeps brutal hours) shows up the next day at 6:00 A.M., looks at the X rays, and wakes up Mr. Heart Attack to tell him he must have sextuple bypass surgery immediately.

An army of hospital personnel descend on Mr. Heart Attack to prepare him for the surgery. Every part of his body is X-rayed several times from every possible direction and the pictures immediately disappear into the X-ray file room never to be seen again. Samples of all existing body fluids are withdrawn with needles, injected into gigantic machines, and scrutinized by orange and purple lasers. In their place, lists of numbers spit from the other end of the machines. Consent forms, exonerating the hospital from all possible outcomes, are signed in quintuplicate. A tall man with a fantastically sharp razor appears out of nowhere and shaves Mr. Heart Attack from head to foot the evening before the operation. Dr. Anesthesia, a cohort of Dr. Heart Surgeon who will put Mr. Heart Attack to sleep, arrives at 3:00 P.M., says hello, and leaves. A battalion of interns—medical interns, surgical interns, anesthesia interns—crawl from the woodwork in the middle of the night, scrutinize Mr. Heart Attack and all of his numbers (as well as his X rays, which they have somehow managed to rescue from the bowels of the X-ray file room), and slither out again. Nurses cajole him and give him a last bath.

The next day, Mr. Heart Attack goes to the operating room. Dr. Cardiothoracic (CT) Surgery Fellow, the guy training to become a big-cheese heart surgeon, and Dr. Fifth-Year Surgeon chop open his chest, attach all the plumbing leading to and from his heart to a heart-lung machine, and then stop the heart. A surgical intern holds metal hooks that keep the operating field clear while the CT surgery fellow and the fifth-year general surgeon hack away. The intern can see nothing of the operating field and tries desperately not to fall asleep on his feet.

Dr. Heart Surgeon struts into the room and everyone salutes. Doc Veins has been busily stripping lengths of vein out of Mr. Heart Attack's legs. The veins are sitting in a bowl. Dr. Heart Surgeon uses the veins to fashion new heart arteries for Mr. Heart Attack, tubes that will replace the ones that have become hopelessly clogged. The procedure takes a half hour. He then reconnects all the plumbing that was attached to the heart-lung machine during the surgery, and shocks the heart to restart it. For the purposes of this story we will assume that the patient doesn't box but actually makes it through the surgery. His heart restarts. Dr. Heart Surgeon leaves and the CT fellow and fifth-year sew closed Mr. Heart Attack's chest.

Mr. Heart Attack goes to the surgical ICU for a few days, where he is again descended upon by dozens of interns and other staff until he is stable enough to go to a regular room. The Drs. Private drop in every day, write a note, and leave. Mr. Heart Attack recovers from his surgery and leaves the hospital.

About ten or fifteen members of the medical and surgical staff have been involved in Mr. Heart Attack's care. They all work 80 to 120 hours a week and, in New York City, earn from $28,000 to $35,000 a year, or $3 to $5 an hour (before taxes). Of every twenty-four hours of Mr. Heart Attack's stay, including that in the OR and intensive care units, a member of the housestaff has been at his side an average of two to five hours.

The nurses and therapists work thirty-six to forty hours a week and earn $21,000 to $35,000 a year, depending on their level of experience, approximately $10 to $15 an hour. While Mr. Heart Attack is in the "expensive care unit" the nurses spend an average of five to nine hours a day with him. The therapists, whose work comes later, will spend an hour or two several times a week with Mr. Heart Attack for the first few weeks after his surgery.

The techs and clerks work a forty-hour week and earn $12,000 to $16,000 a year. During his stay they have devoted three or four hours a day to Mr. Heart Attack's stay.

Dr. Heart Specialist will have spent a total of three to five hours with Mr. Heart Attack for the entire duration of his stay. He'll charge several grand for his services. Dr. Heart Tests, who did the fancy X rays, will charge $750 to $1,500 for his hour's work. Dr. Heart Surgeon, who did the cabbage (coronary artery bypass graft—CABG), and spent a total of a few hours with the patient, will charge ten or fifteen grand. The gas man (anesthesia) will charge a few more. The Drs. Private will charge $25,000 to $35,000 out of a total hospital bill of $50,000 or $75,000.

Now, you tell me, why is the system set up the way it is?

I got a tremendous kick recently from talking to one of the private docs, an internist at MH. He was lamenting recently proposed legislation in New York State that would limit the number of consecutive hours doctors in training work to a maximum of twenty-four.

This legislation was proposed, incidentally, after a recent scandal involving a young drug abuser with a psychiatric history who was accidentally killed by the housestaff at a fancy New York hospital. The junkie's father happened to be a big shot and sued the hospital. In the course of the trial it was revealed that a contributing factor in the accidental death was the fact that the housestaff involved in the patient's care were grossly overworked. Surprise, surprise.

The private doc I was talking to was wearing a silk

jacket, a silk tie, and a gold-plated stethoscope. After a brief discussion about the legislation, an idea that should have been made law decades ago, he asked me, wide-eyed, "I think it's a great idea, but where are they going to get the money?"

I could only laugh.

12

Therapeutic Minimalism

At this point it should be clear that there is a whole hell of a lot more going on in hospitals than patient care. In fact, given the politics, anger, resentment, and craziness, it's a miracle that the patients manage to survive, never mind get better. In addition to being sick, the patient is forced to deal with both iatrogenic and nosocomial causes of illness. To me it became quite obvious that perhaps the best thing to be done for a patient was nothing. The patient is saved the indignities inherent to the hospital and may focus his strength on recovery from the illness that brought about medical attention, or inattention, as the case may be. In medical school my favorite preceptors were of the type called therapeutic minimalists. They believed that the safest management of a patient, especially one in no immediate danger of crashing, was for the doctor to calm down and watch. If a drug had to be used it should be one that had been around a minimum of fifteen or twenty years with proven harmlessness in the long term, and whose use was well known, like penicillin or aspirin.

One evening I admitted a nice woman to Cloud who had intestinal obstruction. She'd shown up in the ER barfing her brains out, totally unable to keep anything down. An X ray of her abdomen established that her guts were blocked. The potential causes were myriad, ranging from the horrible, like a tumor, to nothing at all, a mere temporary work stoppage for unknown reasons on the part of the intestines.

Under orders from my resident I stuck an IV into the patient to provide her with the fluids she was unable to take by mouth, inspected the IV site daily to ensure that it wasn't becoming infected, checked her vital signs, and waited. Being pretty new at the business, I worried that a surgeon might need to come and cut the patient open to manually unblock her tubes. My resident told me to shut up and relax. When the poor lady ran out of veins to stick IVs into I asked about putting in a central line. I was instructed to look for IV sites between her toes before talking about central lines, and I managed to find a spot for the line.

One day, about a week after she was admitted, the patient began to belch and fart like crazy. We sent her for another X ray of her belly and discovered that her intestines had unblocked themselves. I walked into her room and gave her a glass of water to drink. She did so without vomiting it back up into my face, as she had when she was first admitted. She got so excited that she could drink a glass of water again that she started crying and thanking me and slobbering big, wet kisses on my cheeks. Two days later she was able to eat normal food and we discharged her. We had done absolutely nothing for her except give her fluids and let her get better on her own. If we'd actually treated her she'd probably be dead today.

Another example of therapeutic minimalism involved a baby I saw one day in the NYG ER. I was minding my own business, attending to some poor, ill, elderly patient in the "medical-critical area" of the ER (an area set up to attend to the one in fifty patients whose illness actually was an emergency) when the head nurse came barreling in and plunged a baby into my arms.

The nurse and infant, a tiny pink object that appeared perplexed and amused by the noise and commotion, were followed by a very handsome, very stern, very matronly-looking grandmother. Next, with a bright red, flushed face, a white T-shirt, white pants, white apron, and top to bottom coating of white flour, came an uncle, an employee of a nearby bakery. Apparently, he had only moments before come rushing from his place of employment to accompany his niece on her emergency visit to the emergency room. Behind uncle, and shuddering with sobs, was the baby's oh-so-young and pretty mommy, her mascara a mess, her heaving shoulders held firmly and sturdily by her equally young and pretty, and grievously concerned, sister.

All at once all the members of the family began shrieking.

"The baby, the baby, the BABY! Doctor, doctor, DOCTOR! The baby, she's not breathing! The baby, she stopped BREATHING!"

In a situation like this it is the doctor's first duty to remain absolutely and totally calm, and to immediately remove the baby from the emotion-laden family, who are then escorted away to the waiting area. This the head nurse and I accomplished at once. We then took the baby into a private room to examine her. We looked down at her, back up at each other, and again back down at the baby. She gazed up at us, trying to decide whether or not to cry. I put my stethoscope to her back and heard breaths, quiet and rhythmic.

I looked back up at the nurse. "They lied, this baby in actual fact *is* breathing, do you agree?"

She smiled. "Looks that way to me."

I gave the baby a very quick once-over, at which time she immediately elected to cry vigorously. I asked the head nurse to reassure the family that the baby was breathing and then to send the stern-looking grandma in to talk to me.

Grandma told me that the baby had been feeding and she'd choked and stopped breathing, but she wasn't exactly sure what happened because she wasn't there. I asked her to have mom come in.

Mom came in, sniffling with relief and remembered anguish, and I plopped the sobbing baby in her arms. I asked her what happened.

"The baby, I was feeding her and she choked and stopped breathing, is she okay now? Oh my GOD!" She stared down at her rapidly calming infant, horrified.

I assured her that, whatever it was that had happened, the baby was indeed fine now, and then dispatched the entire family to the pediatrics clinic to get a lecture on how to properly position a baby during feeding so that it doesn't choke.

About two hours later the uncle reappeared in the ER, still clad in white cotton and white flour, carrying a half-dozen boxes stuffed full with Italian pastries. He gave a box to each of the nurses and then handed one to me.

"Doctor," he said, "I want to thank you with all my heart. You saved my niece's life."

Of course, there were many patients for whom we had to do something, for whom therapeutic minimalism did not constitute appropriate, decent medical care. There were walking, talking, sick patients, the kind we sincerely wanted to help, patients for whom we did our best, but who, naturally, we only made sicker. There were those whom we tortured mercilessly in the name of good medical care, and who were fortunate to wind up leaving the hospital alive. For those unlucky enough to be nice guys we went all out, breaking our silly-ass necks in the hope our actions would help. And this, of course, was what wound up making things even worse.

The vascular surgery patient, the Diabetic Man Who Came into the Hospital with a Cold Toe, for example, was the classic case of a nice guy who underwent torment, torment, torment all because we were so damn eager to help.

The Diabetic Man Who Came into the Hospital with a Cold Toe was a terrific, charming old guy who'd had a terrible case of diabetes for many years. He was suffering diabetic vascular disease that had severely compromised the circulation to his lower legs. His big toe, deprived of an adequate blood supply, had become cold and blue almost to the point of gangrene.

Now, the patient had two things going against him. Number one, he was a really nice old guy, the kind of guy docs break their necks for. Number two, he was admitted to the hospital by the most aggressive vascular surgeon in the world, a man who just happened to work out of MH, a surgeon named Dr. Schlashman.

Dr. Schlashman behaved as though he was a protégé of Dr. Big over at NYG. He was renowned for ferocious patient advocacy, and for equally ferocious treatment of the housestaff. The surgical residents at MH shuddered at the thought of rotating on the vascular service because they knew it would be a solid month of torture under the aegis of Dr. Schlashman.

A friend of mine who worked on one of the Cloud floors had one of Dr. Schlashman's patients transferred to his service one day. The patient, who'd already had his surgical procedure, developed a complication and Schlashman wanted him "turfed" to the medical people for further care.

The patient had had some kind of vascular graft done on both of his legs, a basic rerouting of blood around diseased blood vessels, designed to improve the circulation of blood to his lower legs. When my friend and his resident showed up to examine the guy, they found him lying in bed wearing a pair of surgical support stockings. Schlashman showed up at the same moment to check up on the patient and, when he saw the surgical stockings, exploded in anger.

"Wha—! Who the FUCK, . . . what kind of FUCK-ING *MEDICAL* ASSHOLE [extra emphasis on "medical" to distinguish the asshole from a surgeon] put a goddam FUCKING pair of stockings on my *goddam* patient!" Dr. Schlashman was perturbed because no patient with a fresh vascular graft in his leg should be wearing a stocking that might lessen the flow of blood.

He turned to the resident, shrieking, "Are you the ASSHOLE who did this?"

The resident, a woman who'd been around awhile, glared back at him. "First of all, I had nothing to do with this patient until two minutes ago, and second of all I don't think that is appropriate language to—"

Schlashman cut her off. "FUCK!! FUCKITY-FUCKITY-FUCK-FUCK and FUCK! Is that the kind of language you're talking about? Well, FUCK YOU, ASSHOLE!" He stomped out of the room.

That was the kind of guy Schlashman was with the housestaff.

With regard to patients, he was renowned for going to every possible extreme to save near gangrenous limbs. He'd done two separate major surgeries on the Diabetic Man Who Came into the Hospital with a Cold Toe to rebuild the arteries in his leg. Both reconstructions had failed to deliver adequate blood to the toe and he reluctantly made the decision to amputate.

Now, amputating a cold blue toe is much more complicated than simply chopping it off. By virtue of the very fact that it is cold and blue it is usually also infected. When an infected limb is amputated the surgeon must always leave the stump open for a few days or a week to ensure that no infected tissue has escaped the knife. If all

213

the flesh at the site of the amputation is healthy, it remains reddish-pink. If there is any infected tissue, it becomes yellow-gray and must be further snipped ("debrided") until the area is clearly healthy and can be sewed closed.

The Diabetic Man had his infected big toe cut off. Dr. Schlashman left the wound open and after a few days yellow stuff appeared, suggesting that he hadn't removed all of the infected tissue. The housestaff gave the patient 50 mg of Demerol for pain, and, using scissors and scalpel blades, scraped off the yellow-and-gray tissue.

After a few more days more yellow-and-gray tissue appeared. The housestaff reappeared with scissors and scalpels and scraped it off, too. A few days later it appeared again so Schlashman decided to cut the patient's foot in half about an inch in front of his toes, a transmetatarsal amputation. He made sure to cut a good inch away from any infected-looking tissue.

He left the wound open and two or three days later more gray-yellow stuff appeared. This was duly debrided and after several more episodes of off-color tissue and debridement, Dr. Schlashman decided to perform a BKA, a below-knee amputation. Careful inspection of this wound soon revealed that the patient's poor debilitated blood vessels were unable to adequately supply the site of the BKA, and it became infected, too.

The Diabetic Man Who Came into the Hospital with a Cold Toe left about two months later, his leg amputated about four inches above the knee, the wound closed and well healed.

The joke goes that there are three guys shipwrecked on an uncharted island somewhere in the Pacific. They are captured by the local natives and tied to posts in the center of the village.

The village chief, resplendent in war paint, approaches the first of the three and says, "You have a choice. You may choose *chu-cha* or you may choose death."

The first sailor thinks to himself, "I don't know what this *chu-cha* is, but I don't want to die," and says, "I'll take *chu-cha*."

The chief says, "You have chosen." He turns to the villagers and cries, "*Chu-cha!!*" The villagers jump up and down and throw themselves on the ground in a frenzy, shaking and pounding the ground with poles topped by shrunken heads, shrieking, "*Chu-cha! Chu-cha! Chu-cha!*"

The first man is taken into a hut and the men of the village mercilessly beat and rape him for hours until he is bleeding and semiconscious. Finally, they drag him out of the hut and dump him on the ground in front of the second, where he emits a last gasp and dies.

The chief stands before the second and says, "You have a choice, you may choose *chu-cha*, or you may choose death."

The second man is horrified but thinks, "Well, this is really bad, but maybe . . . well, maybe I'm a little tougher than he was, maybe I'll survive this *chu-cha*."

He looks at the chief and says, "I'll take *chu-cha*."

The chief says, "You have chosen," turns to the villagers, and cries, "*Chu-cha!*" The villagers again throw themselves to the ground, frenzied, and shriek, "*Chu-cha! Chu-cha! Chu-cha!*"

The second sailor disappears into the hut and when he is dragged out hours later and dumped in front of the third man he is already dead.

The chief stands before the third man and says, "What is your choice?" and the man immediately says, "Death!"

The chief turns back to the villagers and says, "He has chosen. Death by *chu-cha!!!*"

* * *

215

The Diabetic Man Who Came into the Hospital with a Cold Toe had all the appropriate medical care. He had the grafts in hopes of saving his toe, the amputation of his toe in hopes of saving his foot, the trans-met in hopes of saving his lower leg, the BKA in hopes of saving the function of his knee. He'd been treated well and appropriately, he'd had the most advanced care medicine had to offer, and what he got was five months of *chu-cha*.

There may be people who read this and think I'm being a little bit too pessimistic. It's true that I've emphasized the more negative aspect of my medical experience. I'll admit that there is the occasional instance of someone getting better, even when the doctor isn't a therapeutic minimalist. I've done a fair amount of actively intervening (an "active intervention" is medical jargon for actually doing something for a patient). This is sometimes necessary with people who are very sick, or potentially very sick.

One large class of the very sick are the very sick, very old, and very demented (very "senile"). I respect the very old, in fact I try to respect everyone (even junkies), and do my best for all my patients, old or not, demented or not. That's my job. And, on rare occasions, I am successful. Nonetheless, it is more satisfying to help those who have at least a little bit of spunk. Active intervention, "doing my best," for those who spend twenty-four hours a day pretzeled up in bed staring numbly at the sheets is often frustrating. It sometimes seems unfair to torment people for whom life offers little more than torture in the hospital.

Oldness, incidentally, is a function of sickness, and not the other way around. I've seen a number of walking, talking people over the age of one hundred who were much healthier than their sixty-year-old grandchildren. A little gentle intervention for these people can be very

216

satisfying.

Another large class of the very sick are people with cancer, heart disease, and lung disease. A tremendous amount of intervening can be done for someone having a heart attack. Because such a patient usually comes under the walking, talking category, making the pain of heart attack go away can be satisfying, too. The same goes for helping people with lung problems breathe better. Helping people breathe better is my favorite medical intervention.

I have mixed feelings about cancer, especially the particularly vicious types like lung tumors. I understand why people who have cancer want to be treated. In fact, I understand it very well. The alternative is death, and to subject oneself to the horror of cancer treatment as a stand against death is certainly logical. Unfortunately, much cancer treatment does little more than transform the final years, months, or weeks of an individual's life into a period of unnecessary pain. Often it hastens death. Given that the last months or weeks of someone's life can be a period of reflection, love, and reconciliation, this outcome is particularly tragic. For many, the tragedy of cancer treatment is the failure to attend to the emotional and social needs of the patient, needs that become especially acute in cancer, as well as the medical details. As was the case with Mr. Smith, many cancer patients become little more than ravaged medical battlegrounds.

In the best of circumstances people are treated for vicious illness in the hopes that treatment will prolong life without too great a cost in torment, in the hopes that the time granted a patient through treatment will be "quality time." Nonetheless, it is frustrating to realize that most wouldn't get so sick if Americans didn't smoke or eat shitty food. As a doc I have gotten to feeling like a less than significant bandage for a society that refuses to behave responsibly. It's like the army recruiting doctors to work at the front. The need would be obviated were

217

people simply to refuse to send their children to fight in wars.

I finally decided that the most important thing I could possibly do for anybody was to keep them the hell out of the hospital. The hospital had proved to be such a prime cause of human carnage that I believed this to be virtually my foremost duty.

The best opportunity to achieve this end arose in clinic, where I saw a number of patients, regulars of mine, and did my best to keep them from being admitted.

In this spirit I dragged entire families into my office to give them long and detailed lectures about how to treat an ill family member at home, people who would much more easily be dumped in the hospital. I even gave people my home phone number in case they needed to call and ask a question in the middle of the night. I sent ailing little old ladies like Mrs. Guttierez home to bed, trailed by children and cousins and spouses armed with lists of tasks, medication doses and times, and prescriptions. I sent coughing, vomiting, feverish babies back to the safety of their cribs, their mommies and daddies loaded with babies' Tylenol, ampicillin tablets, and complicated feeding and care instructions. I drew blood cultures in the clinic, ready to rocket the patient into the hospital at the slightest hint of one becoming positive.

One of the patients I visited at home on at least a quasi-regular basis was a lady in her mid-sixties who was ravaged by diabetes. Diabetes is a vicious disease and Gloria had all of its vicious outcomes. She'd lost both legs to diabetic vascular disease and was wheelchair-bound in a three-story walk-up apartment. I visited her at home because having no legs made getting to the clinic an enormous production for her. I asked her to come in only once or twice a year when it couldn't be helped, like when she needed an electrocardiogram or a chest X ray, things that couldn't be done at home.

Gloria became my patient at about the middle of my internship year, and I continued to look after her for the rest of my training. She was a regular of mine, like my friend Mr. Martinez, the junkie homosexual who was neglected to death during an admission for fever. I really enjoyed going to Gloria's house because she lived on a real solid Italian block downtown. After a while I got to know the locals by sight. Wearing my shirt and tie, I rode a motorcycle to get to Gloria's apartment, much to the amusement of the people who hung around on the stoop in front of her building. I never bothered to lock up the bike because I knew the people on the street would keep an eye on it for me.

Gloria had a hell of a case of diabetes. In addition to her amputated legs she had kidney disease that would eventually necessitate dialysis to make her pee for her, congestive heart failure, angina, diabetic eye disease that rendered her legally blind, neuropathy causing pain and numbness in both of her hands, and high blood pressure. She was about as chronically ill as it's possible to get and all of her illness was related to diabetes.

Gloria and I spent a few years doing what I called chasing numbers. Being a doctor, I was very number-oriented and targeted each of her various problems, at least those that could be measured numerically, to specific "normal limits." Blood pressure, blood glucose (sugar), fat, and cholesterol; all could be reduced to numbers. One week her blood pressure would be totally out of control while her blood sugar was within a few hundred points of normal, while the next the reverse would be true.

Gloria's most impressive numbers were generated by fat and cholesterol. She had so much fat and cholesterol in her veins that her blood plasma, the portion of blood remaining after all the red cells are removed, usually watery, clear, and straw-colored, was actually white and creamy, like milk. I'd send a specimen of her blood to the lab two or three times a year, and then march around the clinic and amaze my friends when the result came back. They all had different ideas about what to do to fix it, with some suggesting medication and others that Gloria's diet be changed. I had no faith that any of the anticholesterol medications fit into the category of "drugs that actually work," and bullied her relentlessly about the food she ate. I even showed up unannounced at her apartment to snoop around in the refrigerator, looking for fatty foods. Although the worst I'd ever find was a box of cookies, her plasma continued to look like heavy cream. Finally, I relented on the idea of medicine and looked up one of the cholesterol-lowering drugs in the *Physician's Desk Reference*. I discovered that the World Health Organization had done a study on the drug, showing that more people had died of its side effects than were saved by its cholesterol-lowering effects. I closed the book and called Gloria to remind her to keep her diet.

In reality, Gloria's numbers didn't make a whole lot of difference to her. The things that did make a difference, that she had no legs, couldn't see, and had hands that hurt all the time, were the aspects of her illness that, naturally, I could do nothing about.

Gloria visited the eye clinic twice a month for diabetic eye disease, and the eye doc blasted the tiny bleeding blood vessels in her retinas (the back of the eye) with a laser. Although this bleeding was the cause of her progressive loss of sight, the laser treatments could only slow the process, and eventually she would become completely blind. Photos of her retinas, which showed the blood vessels dotted with laser burns, looked like aerial reconnaissance photos of German cities after World War II bombing raids. Gloria fought with me constantly, demanding to know, "Why the hell should I drag myself in for treatments that leave me seeing spots for two days if I'm going to go blind anyhow." It was an understandable argument.

As with her failing vision, the tingling, numbness, and pain in Gloria's hands was a problem I could do little about. The result of a little understood effect of diabetes on nerves, diabetic neuropathy had destroyed her ability to do any kind of detailed work with her hands, including relatively simple tasks like turning a key in a keyhole. I read all the up-to-date literature, tried a few esoteric drugs, referred Gloria to neurologists, and even had her fitted with a little transistor radio-sized box that was supposed to help by shooting low-voltage currents of electricity into her hands, but nothing did any good.

Gloria's worst problem was her breathing. She had a terrible case of congestive heart failure. Her heart, once a strong pumping muscle, had become swollen, baggy, and tired, just like Mr. Kram's, my ancient sundowner on Cloud. This also was the result of the ravages of diabetes on blood vessels (in this particular case, the blood vessels that supplied the heart muscle with oxygen and nutrients). Diabetes had successfully attacked just about all of the blood vessels in Gloria's body.

Gloria's lungs often got so wet from the fluid that backed up behind her congested heart that she'd be unable to do anything but sit in her wheelchair and gasp for breath, turning bluer and bluer until she was finally forced to call an ambulance to take her to the emergency room. The emergency room doctor, placing his stethoscope on her back, would hear her lungs sloshing around in two or three liters of extra fluid, bubbling noisily with each breath. He'd plug an IV in her arm, make her pee like a bandit with Lasix, and after she'd peed off a few liters, enough to dry out her lungs and relieve her short-

221

ness of breath, he'd send her home. Sometimes she was in such bad shape on arrival in the ER that she had to be admitted for a few days, and then my quest to keep her out of the hospital had failed.

Gloria and a few of her family members had lived on the same street for the past thirty or forty years. She could tell who people were just by the sound they made when they opened the front door to her building, three floors below. One of her favorite activities was to attend gigantic family feasts that were held in celebration of various Italian holidays. Her big, burly, tattooed brothers and nephews would come and trundle her off in her wheelchair to the site of these gatherings, and she'd load up on sausage and peppers and the like, salty food all. This, of course, was the absolute worst thing for her congestive heart failure, and she'd get bloated with salty fluid that eventually found its way to her lungs. More than once a family feast was culminated by an unexpected visit to the emergency room.

When a holiday was near I'd tell her, "Listen Gloria, I can't blame you if you want to eat a decent meal, but do yourself and me a favor and take an extra Lasix or two before you eat, so that you don't wind up back in the ER at MH." She was on a standing dose of Lasix that kept her fluids in a precarious balance. What she peed off balanced what she took in, preventing her from becoming overloaded with fluid. The added salt and water she'd take on at holidays could be offset simply by bumping up the dose and making her pee more.

Sometimes this worked and sometimes it didn't. Gloria was taking a lot of medicine, about twenty pills a day (when I started seeing her she was taking closer to forty a day; we spent the first two months taking her off of medications to get down to twenty), and was naturally a little skittish about messing around with the doses. After a series of Catholic holiday feasts followed by emergency room visits I learned to be more specific. I'd say, "I want you to take one extra ten-mg Lasix pill for every helping of sausage and pepper," and her lungs would stay dry as a bone.

Before the discovery of insulin, diabetes was a uniformly fatal disease. The blood of the diabetic became superconcentrated by extremely high levels of sugar and the by-products of fat metabolism, and the kidneys, unable to excrete a fluid so concentrated, allowed the loss of large volumes of water. The diabetic eventually became unable to keep up with the cycle of massive thirst and drinking, and an almost constant need to urinate, and died of dehydration.

Today, by injecting natural or synthetic insulin, the diabetic is able to utilize the glucose in his blood and never develops the high concentrations that formerly killed people (and occasionally still do). Now, the more long-term and insidious consequences of diabetes, particularly its destructive effects on the body's small blood vessels (the "microvasculature"), have time to develop. Almost all of Gloria's problems, such as blindness, congestive heart failure, kidney disease, and neuropathy, were the result of decades of diabetic vascular disease.

Gloria was on 70 units of insulin a day when I started seeing her. Although this is enough to cause hypoglycemia (low blood sugar) in a bull elephant, it didn't keep her in good control. Her blood glucose ranged from 400 to 700 (normal is 80-120), high enough to make the average internist break out in a sweat. It seemed to me that the logical response was to increase the insulin, and after a year I had her on over 80 units daily, a truly industrial-strength dose. Naturally, her sugars got even worse. Finally, I decided to try decreasing the dose instead, and seeing if that might help. A few months later her glucose was under 200 at 30 units a day. I'm sure that a diabetologist could explain this, but I've no idea why it worked.

Diet is an important part of the control of diabetes, and

223

sausage and peppers were not the only troublemaker foods that Gloria enjoyed at holidays. No feast was complete without a platter laden with sugary pastries—cannolis, Italian cheesecakes, rum cakes—all potential causes of record-setting glucose levels. I'd ask Gloria to increase the insulin dose if she was going to indulge herself, say 5 extra units for every rum cake, and 8 for a cannoli. Strange how the dates of Italian Catholic *festas* were so important to Gloria's medical care, how they acted as warning lights for her dietary indiscretions. During Lent her glucose and fluids were well controlled, but, when Christ ascended, so did her insulin and Lasix.

Sometimes Gloria feared a drop in glucose to too *low* a level, and refused to play with the insulin dose. Also, her eye problem made it difficult for her to read the tiny numbers on the insulin syringes and she feared an accidental overdose. Then, when she ate something sugary, she'd get panicked and confused and call the man from the commercial blood test laboratory to come and draw her blood. I'd plead with her not to do this, but she did so several times anyway, using her Medicaid card to pay for the service. Then, when she got the results she'd call me in a panic.

She'd wail into the phone, "I don't know what happened. My sugar is six-fifty. Whaddamy gonna do?"

A blood glucose of 650 is quite impressive, impressive enough to cause a sweaty internist to hospitalize a diabetic patient for treatment and control.

I'd say, "Well, how did it get so high? The last time it was checked it was around three hundred." Three hundred is also a value that raises an internist's hackles, but it wasn't until later, when we discovered the paradoxical effect of lower insulin doses, that her sugars started to come down near normal.

Gloria would reply, "I don't know. I didn't do anything to raise it up. These goddam needles ain't doing nothing

224

and I'm going to go off 'em."

I knew she wouldn't go through with such a threat because, as terrible as the needles were, she needed them to stay alive and she knew it.

I'd say, "Listen, Gloria, I told you it was okay to have dessert every once in a while so long as you raised the insulin five or ten units. If you're going to stop taking the needles then you know you're going to have to keep your diet. How about you do that for a few days and then have the sugar rechecked?"

After three days of rigorously keeping her diet, and not one extra drop of insulin, she'd have the man return with his needles and test tubes to redraw her blood. More often than not, her sugar would drop several hundred points.

In retrospect I realize that the three years I spent visiting Gloria at home meant very little in comparison with the overall duration of her illness. She'd had diabetes for over twenty years and would continue to have it long after I finished my training and left MH. Years earlier she'd been attended by one of the old community docs, a man who'd looked after her for decades before dying of cancer. Gloria was the kind of patient who required total dedication from a doctor, the kind of doctor who devoted a lifetime to medicine, to a group of patients, a hospital, and a community.

13

Death

I was close to twenty years old before I first saw a dead person. This happened when I was a volunteer in the ER at the Bronx Borough Hospital (BBH), a fateful period after my first year of college when, flushed and eager, I decided medicine was an ideal way to make my contribution to mankind. I specifically and vividly remember looking at my first dead patient and thinking about him, although I don't remember at all what had happened to him or how he had wound up dead in the ER.

The strange thing, looking back on it, was his being dead (dead and cold, as he'd been dead for some time) and fully dressed. He was lying on a stretcher with the curtain drawn, nobody paying attention to him at all, and I just stood and looked at him for a while. It was strange that he was fully dressed because most dead patients have their clothes cut off by doctors and nurses during the code, the attempt to bring them back to life. For this reason virtually everybody who is declared dead in the ER winds up naked as well as dead. Naked at the moment of birth and naked at the moment of death.

I can't imagine, in retrospect, why my first dead person was allowed to remain dressed for his passage into the next world. Perhaps he arrived so clearly dead that the ER staff gave him a break and decided not to code him. Perhaps the chief medical resident was in the ER at the time and said, "How about we leave this one be, for once? He's clearly been dead for a while now, so whaddaya say we leave well enough alone?" and everybody agreed, so they left him dead with all his clothes on.

I distinctly remember his being clothed because he had a pair of glasses in a vinyl case in his breast pocket. Had he been coded his glasses would certainly have landed on the floor, followed by cut-up clothes, blood, and garbage. The glasses made the fact that the dead man was recently alive much more real for me. The dead man had glasses in his pocket because only hours earlier he'd had a use for them and reached for them, probably for reading the paper or doing other up-close work with his eyes. To me this meant he'd just been alive. Were he dressed up in a coffin in a funeral home they wouldn't put the glasses in his breast pocket. This would look ridiculous. Dead people in funeral homes are dressed for death, not life, and they have no need for the paraphernalia of life, things like reading glasses.

But, in the ER, the man was so close to life that he still had his glasses in his pocket. I stood for a while looking at the man and these thoughts led to other thoughts, about who he was and what he was like and that kind of thing.

It's now quite a few years later, about ten or twelve or something like that, though it's much more a distance of mind than of years between now and when I first saw that dead man in the ER. Although there must be a register somewhere in my brain of every single dead person I've seen since then, the exact number eludes my conscious memory. It's probably in the neighborhood of 250 to 500. I've helped code 100 or 150 dead folks, acted as primary doc for 25 to 50 people who wound up dead while in my care, notified 40 to 60 family members of a patient's demise, and actually seen 5 or 6 people make the transition from awake, aware, and alert to dead, dead, and dead.

In medicine, cessation of heartbeat and breathing constitute "clinical death." Clinically dead people are "coded" (a procedure, as I've mentioned, more properly referred to as "advanced cardiac life support," involving chest massage, artificial respiration, and the administration of fancy drugs that I'll describe in horrifying detail later) in an attempt to restore breathing lungs and beating hearts.

That death can be "clinical" suggests other kinds of death; and, indeed, there is also "biological" death. Biological death describes the actual dying of the tissues of the body, from lack of oxygen, rather than mere cessation of heartbeat and respirations. Interestingly, different parts of the body have different capacities to survive without oxygen. Arms and legs, for example, do better than viscera like intestines and kidneys, which do better than the brain and heart. Arms and legs can go an hour or more without oxygen before they become totally and irreversibly dead.

In terms of the patient's eventual recovery after an episode of clinical death, the brain and heart are the limiting factor, the weak link in the chain. A patient who remains pulseless and without respirations for more than five minutes tends to die irreversibly. A medical team could pump on him for weeks, but he'd never recover.

One of the patients whose death I witnessed was a woman who had a very large heart attack one night while she was out eating dinner with her husband. She was rushed by ambulance from the restaurant to the ER at Manhattan Hospital where, over a period of an hour, her heart failed almost completely.

On arrival at the hospital she was the picture of a massive heart attack complicated by low blood pressure and all the medical students gathered around to watch as we started to do all the things necessary for such a patient.

A heart attack, very plainly put, is the result of a blockage of the coronary arteries, the tubes that supply blood, with its load of oxygen and nutrients, to the pumping muscle of the heart itself. If a heart attack is small, the loss of muscle is not great enough to compromise the heart's action as a pump. If it is "massive," the loss of a large chunk of muscle causes it to fail as a pump, and blood pressure falls. In medical lingo, shock caused by a failing heart is called cardiogenic shock.

Our first step in the patient's management was to put an oxygen mask on her face. By increasing the amount of oxygen she breathed, more would enter the blood for delivery to her straining heart. Next we would attempt to raise her blood pressure, and further improve the flow of blood and oxygen to her heart muscle by using fluids and medications. We stuck several IV lines into her veins to give fluid to expand her blood volume. Administering volume in this way is often done to people in shock. The reasoning is that increasing the amount of the blood is one logical way to increase blood pressure. In traumatic shock, low blood pressure resulting from loss of blood after a gunshot wound, stabbing, car accident, or whatever, IVs are used to pour in bags and bags of blood that people have donated to the blood bank. Hopefully, such donated blood is free of the AIDS virus, and successfully replaces that lost through the trauma (which is repaired by surgeons).

Unfortunately, volume often doesn't help in shock that is caused by an attacked, failing heart because it doesn't matter how much blood there is if the heart can't pump it. Also, administering fluid can complicate the congestion that occurs as blood backs up behind the failing heart. Rather than raising blood pressure, the fluid dribbles out into the billions of little tiny air bags in the lungs, just as it did in poor old Mr. Kram as I chased fluid into and out of his lungs during his stay on Cloud. When fluid is given in cardiogenic shock, it must be administered in small amounts, with frequent checks to ensure that the lungs aren't being flooded.

Morphine, one of the top ten "drugs that actually work," can have dramatic effects in both heart attacks and heart failure. By helping take away the pain and anxiety that accompany a heart attack, morphine helps the heart relax, lessening its need for oxygen. It is useful in cardiogenic shock because it can help relieve the buildup of fluid in the lungs. On the other hand, morphine can also lower blood pressure, a big no-no in shock. It is chemically related to Demerol, the stuff I used to sedate and almost kill the poor ninety-five-year-old asthmatic lady whom I'd tubed at NYG when she got too tired to breathe. Like "volume," morphine has to be used very carefully and in small amounts in cardiogenic shock. Both measures are classic double-edged swords that can easily finish off an already critically ill patient.

We gave the lady a dollop of IV fluid and a smidgen of morphine and she felt a little bit better. Her husband was present, complete with stains on his tie from the dinner he'd been eating with his wife before she started to die. He looked like he was in layperson's shock so we asked him to sit down in the emergency room waiting area. After a while we sent a medical student to talk to him who said, "We gave your wife some medicine and she's feeling a little better," a blatant lie told so that he also might feel a little better.

There is a saying in medicine, "The truth is what is best for the patient." If, after a great deal of thinking, it is apparent that a lie might be better for a patient than the truth, it is okay to go ahead and tell it. Most people will think this is another example of doctors playing God, but it isn't. Such lying is not to be taken lightly or with little thought, and it should be of clear benefit to the patient.

For example, if a man having terrible chest pain, fear, and anxiety from a big-time heart attack asks what is happening and is told the truth, "Well, Mr. Big-time Heart

Attack, you're having a really big-time heart attack and there's a fair chance you're going to die from it," he'll have been done a terrible disservice. He will get more fearful and anxious, his heart will beat even harder and the pain and risk of death will get worse.

On the other hand, he may be told a lie. "Well, sir, it looks like you may be having a heart problem but we'll have no trouble at all getting rid of the pain, and besides even if it is a heart attack it really doesn't look too bad." If these words help the patient relax and feel less pain the fact that they weren't true is of little significance. Words, phrases, gestures, even the touch of a hand, can be therapeutic. Thus, it is important to maintain a calm demeanor in situations like this, even when thinking, "Christ, it looks like this guy is going to kick off just when I was about to get some lunch."

The truth was, the patient did look a tiny bit better, meaning that she still looked absolutely terrible. I sat her up to listen to her lungs after her dollop of IV fluid and heard a symphony of bubbles and crackles, like the sound cellophane makes if you ball it up next to your ear. This was the sound of fluid merrily seeping into her lungs, and it prompted me to reach over and shut off the flow of fluid into her veins. I then got a BP cuff to check if the fluid had helped raise her blood pressure. It hadn't.

I leaned over and whispered in her ear, "Don't worry, Mrs. Kelly, I know you feel very sick but we're going to take good care of you." I didn't add that she looked to have an even shot or better at dying. The truth is what is best for the patient.

Since the fluid hadn't helped raise the patient's blood pressure we next decided to give her a "vasoactive" drug, one that would act directly on the heart to make it beat faster and stronger, directly and emphatically raising her blood pressure. Unfortunately, by making the heart work harder it would also increase its need for oxygen. Vasoac-

231

tive drugs (of which there are several types) are a mixed blessing in cardiogenic shock.

The combination of oxygen and drugs resulted in the patient looking just slightly better. We sent the medical student back out to the waiting area to talk with the woman's husband, Mr. Kelly, who was staring dully at a game show on the big color television set up high on the wall.

He said, "We've given your wife several medications, and she's looking a bit better. I'll keep you informed on how she is doing."

Next, we stuck a needle into the woman's wrist in search of the radial artery, whose arterial blood would be measured in the lab for its oxygen content. Arterial blood, freshly replenished with oxygen from its recent stop at the lungs, is the best place to inquire as to whether a patient is doing a proper job of breathing. The results suggested that the patient's lungs were doing an awful job of getting oxygen into her blood, so we peered down her throat with a flashlight, stuck a plastic endotracheal tube into her windpipe, and hooked her up to a respirator capable of pumping 100-percent-pure oxygen. After waiting a few minutes we again stuck a needle into her wrist, drew out another sample of arterial blood, and sent it for oxygen measurement to determine whether the machine was doing a better job of breathing than were her lungs. The results showed that this was indeed the case.

Despite our blatant and careful lying, the patient by this time had caught on that she wasn't doing too well. The tube in her windpipe prevented her from being able to talk, and she repeatedly grabbed my hand and looked at me with pleading, frightened eyes. I'd bend over to tell her what we were doing, saying, for example, "Mrs. Kelly, you're having a bit of trouble with your breathing so we've put this tube in your throat to help you. Just try to relax and let it breathe for you."

Though the truth is what is best for the patient, the critically ill usually see through hollow reassurances to the blunt reality of their situation. For this patient, the tip-off was probably the endotracheal tube and respirator. She was smart enough to realize we'd tubed her because she was failing at breathing on her own, and knew this meant she was good and sick. I thought about sedating her but knew this was out because of her low blood pressure. She'd be awake and alert, sitting front and center at her own death.

Having done all we could for the patient in the emergency room, we decided to take her up to the coronary care unit (CCU). The breathing machine was removed and a balloonlike device attached to the end of the endotracheal tube. An intern stood at the head of the stretcher squeezing the balloon rhythmically, mimicking the action of the respirator. Now unencumbered of the large machine, several interns, residents, and medical students eased the patient along on her gurney, the rhythmic squeeze and relax, squeeze and relax, squeeze and relax of the manual balloon trailing off in the quiet late night corridor.

In the CCU the patient was transferred from the gurney to a bed. The CCU cared for many people who were intubated and couldn't talk, and the nurses helped them communicate with a list of common questions attached to a clipboard. The patient pointed to the question he wanted answered, for example, "I'm cold, please bring a blanket," "I want to see my doctor," "Where am I?" "I would like to see my husband (wife, relative)," and even, "The question I want to ask is not here. Please bring me a pencil and paper." A few wise-ass interns had added several questions to the bottom of the list like, "I want to see my lawyer," "Please bring me a pizza," and "Please send a nurse who is not fat." Before showing the list to a patient the staff folded the bottom so that these questions were not visible.

I brought the clipboard to the patient's bedside. She

pointed to, "Where am I?" which I answered, and then to, "I would like to see my husband."

We'd guided the increasingly disheveled Mr. Kelly to the tiny family waiting area, the same room in which I'd spoken to Mrs. Pregnant, the daughter of the Lady with Lung Cancer. The room had a TV, a few grimy couches and chairs, and the eternal smell of stale cigarette smoke. I went there to find him wandering around in circles, mumbling to himself, and whisked him into the CCU for a quick visit with his wife. Since Mrs. Kelly could not talk, she and her husband just held hands and cried and, after about five minutes, I whisked Mr. Kelly back out to the family waiting area.

The patient's blood pressure was still way too low. We'd done everything possible with medications so we decided to send for the cardiothoracic surgery fellow to come over and give Mrs. Kelly an intra-aortic balloon pump. This device is a balloon, inserted into the femoral artery in the thigh, and pushed up into the aorta, right next to the heart. It inflates after the heart beats and gives the blood an extra push, helping raise blood pressure. Just before the heart beats again the balloon deflates so as not to work against its action. It reinflates after the next beat, and so on.

Cardiologists have shown that this rather simple device can help people in cardiogenic shock. If the balloon pump doesn't work the patient's only chance at survival is to be rushed off to the operating room where the old failing heart is cut out and replaced by one of those new-fangled plastic jobs from Louisville, Kentucky, or better yet by a human one freshly snatched out of a young motorcycle accident victim (the transplant surgeons who do such work call motorcycles "donor-cycles").

An amazing thing happened while the surgeon was putting in the pump. A fly that had been buzzing around the room while he was working landed directly, right smack on the balloon part of the balloon pump. People were so flab-

234

bergasted at first that no one said anything and then everyone laughed all at once. The $500 balloon pump (or maybe it was $1,500), having been contaminated by little tiny bits of shit from the fly's feet, had to be tossed out and replaced by a new one. The $500 fly. I don't think anyone even managed to swat it after it flew away. I have gone out of my way to kill flies ever since this happened. It is my feeling that they should pay for it as a species, and I'll stop when I've reached $500 worth.

The surgeon put a clean balloon pump into the patient and her blood pressure increased. We invited Mr. Kelly back in for a quick visit though he could barely fit into the room with all the fancy medical machines crowded around his wife: the machine to breathe for her, the machine controlling the inflation and deflation of the balloon pump, the machine recording the rhythm of her heart, machines to pump medications into the IV lines, and a machine to record her blood pressure. The only machine missing was a cash register, which would have tabbed up about $400 an hour. Intern's slang for intensive care unit is "expensive care unit."

Squeezing past all the machines, Mr. Kelly managed to reach his wife's bedside. Since she still could not say anything they again merely held hands and gazed at each other. I figured there should have been another clipboard for occasions like this, with messages like, "I love you," "Tell the kids I love them," and "Don't forget to feed the dog when you get home."

After a few minutes we ushered Mr. Kelly back out of the room. He staggered back to the family waiting area mumbling, "Machines! I never saw so many machines in my life!" It seemed that all the machines were in some way comforting to him.

The patient stabilized and I managed to get a few hours of sleep that night. I slept lying in a fetal position on one of the short couches in the family waiting area. Mr. Kelly spent the night sleeping sitting up on the couch across from me. Both of us inhaled the smell of stale cigarette smoke into our nostrils, hastening the day when we, too, would wind up in the hospital surrounded by machines.

The next day was the do-or-die day for the patient. Although all medications and machines help keep patients alive, they can't be kept on forever and eventually must be "weaned off." The medicines are slowly lowered and the machines turned down in the hope that enough healing has occurred that the heart and lungs can resume their old duties unassisted.

This would be the die day for our patient. While sitting at the nurses' station I heard a racket coming from the patient's room. I walked in to see her clutching at her chest with one hand and knocking things off the bedside table with the other, looking for the clipboard and pencil.

I said, "Are you having chest pain?" and she nodded her head furiously. I handed her the pencil and paper and she wrote, "Will I die?" threw the clipboard on the floor, grabbed my tie with one hand and my hand with the other, and pulled me down about two inches from her face, now running with sweat. Her eyes were brilliant, shiny, and intense and mine were half open and bloodshot and I said, "No, you're not going to die." I glanced up at the heart rhythm monitor and saw that her heart had started to go completely bananas just like she had. She wouldn't let go of my tie so I yelled, "Could I please have some help in here?" and a bunch of nurses and residents rushed in. They started doing things all at once but I couldn't do anything at all because the patient had me by the tie and the hand. I tried but was unable to force her to let go. I kept looking at the heart monitor and finally her heart developed a totally erratic rhythm and her blood pressure dropped to zero. With this she lost all of her strength, let go of my tie and hand, and her arms dropped onto the bed. We spent about a half hour trying to get her heart going again but couldn't, and that was one of the few times I saw someone go from alive and awake and alert to dead, dead, and dead.

14

The Code

In the hospital, death is an inevitability. No matter how skilled and diligent the staff, or well equipped the facility, a certain percentage of patients will die. Death is a constant. What varies from doctor to doctor, hospital to hospital, state to state, and country to country is the management of patients who have died in the hospital.

In New York City, where I trained, the management of in-hospital death is very aggressive. Unless a very well-defined understanding has been arranged among the patient, his private doctor, and the medical housestaff that so called "heroic measures" not be performed, dead people are almost uniformly "coded" when they die. As I've briefly mentioned, this is the process of trying to restore a pulse and blood pressure to the "clinically" dead. The word "code" probably arises from hospitals' use of different code words or phrases over the public address system to direct medical personnel to the bedside of a dead person. Remember, euphemism and discretion are the rule in the hospital when the subject is death, especially in the presence of patients or their families. A straightforward "Dead patient, Four North! Dead patient, Four North!" is considered less than appropriate for blaring up and down the hospital corridors. Instead, vague, shrouded phrases are urgently uttered over the loudspeakers, like "Code Blue, Four North!" or "Team One, Four North!" Phrases replete with jargon but clearly understood by medical and lay people alike. In this fashion, death is treated like a widely known dirty little secret. It is unspeakable but ever present, unseen but everywhere.

At Manhattan Hospital codes were announced with the phrase, "Attention, attention, attention! CAC Cloud Three! CAC Cloud Three!" For years I thought "CAC" stood for "cardiac arrest code" until a friend told me it was meant to be a warning, "Clear all corridors." There was a young guy whose duty was to drop everything when a code was called, grab the "code cart," a big rolling stretcher with a mechanical chest compressor and drawers full of drugs, and go careening down the halls pushing it ahead of him, a madman unleashed. On hearing him coming, staff and family alike flattened themselves up against the walls in hopes of not being run over. Also flying down the hallway was the medical "code team," one of the resident/intern teams on long call. Any of these barreling individuals might knock someone over who'd then sue the hospital; thus the warning, "Clear all corridors!"

The code is an increasingly familiar part of television hospital dramas. The public knows well the harried- and concerned-looking intern shouting such medically inept and incorrect phrases as "He's flatline! Let's shock him!" Suffice it to say that if I ever shocked a patient who was flatline I'd have a good chance of spending the rest of my medical career doing physical exams for an insurance company in Akron, Ohio.

Hollywood's depiction of a code varies dramatically from reality. The code is often more a social than a medical event, especially if occurring late at night when interns gather about the dead person and exchange banter on the night's progress while doing chest compressions. The scene usually centers on a grievously ill and frail patient who has been headed down the tubes for some time. Nine out of ten codes I've attended were simply the final event in an unwavering progression of total body failure. Reasonably, once the patient's lungs, kidneys, intestines, and brains are gone, and his body has become an enormous culture dish for some particularly vicious and virulent hospital-borne bacterial mutant, his heart will also throw in the towel. Admittedly, "sudden cardiac death" is seen with some frequency in the middle-aged man with heart disease who is otherwise relatively well. In fact, because the problem is usually limited to the heart in such patients, they are the ideal candidates for coding, and many actually "survive the code."

Nonetheless, for most, death is not the result of a sudden fit of cardiac anxiety, but the dying of the last embers, bankruptcy and foreclosure after years of fighting creditors, the overrunning of the last bunkers of resistance. And, because the heart does not operate in a vacuum but is part of a complex, interdependent network, the code is very rarely of any benefit to the critically ill, multisystem-failure patient. No matter how hard it is pushed, what meds are given, what voltage of electricity blasts through it, the heart cannot be forced to function when the rest of the body is already dead.

Most often, the victim of the code is an older person who has been in the hospital for some time, like Mr. Smith or the little old lady cared for by Charlie Miller, who slowly gets sicker and sicker, weaker and weaker, until death finally comes wandering by. This unfortunate older person, a person who probably has not had as much attention in years, is suddenly surrounded by a dozen recent teenagers who pump, poke, stab, stick, cut, prod, and abuse him into oblivion. Interns with some resignation inquire of their cointerns whether their night is proving to be a busy one, which inevitably it is, and comment on the difficulty of completing one's work while being a member of the code team. Medical students love the color and movement inherent in codes and are encouraged to "practice their chest compressions." The more aggressive interns busy themselves in the ritualistic placement of a central line, a practice less controlled under the conditions of a code than in the living patient. Highly macho pencil-sized needles are thrust repeatedly into the patient's not necessarily sterile neck until the jugular vein or, fairly frequently, the carotid artery is pierced. No matter which, hundreds of cc of blood, dark and turbid, spills, joining the sweat and vomit smeared all over the patient, the sheets, and the floor.

Since the patient is old, frail, and brittle, ribs snap under the weight of chest compressions. This is accompanied by an audible crack and the sudden appearance of a sickened look on the medical student's face. The nurses, old, jaded hands at codes, bluster about procedural indiscretions and demand that one person and one person only "run" the code (that is, instruct the staff on what meds to give, when to shock the heart, and when to end the code). For the head nurse interpersonal decorum is foremost and the abrupt or rude house officer is likely to lose more patients than the soft-toned resident who liberally sprinkles even-toned med orders with plenty of "pleases" and "thank yous."

Maintaining this appropriately low but in-charge profile is the most senior of the housestaff present, usually a third-year medical resident. Standing next to the electrocardiogram machine, the doc attempts to interpret the paper strip recording of the sputtering, dazed, and chaotic electrical activity of the dying heart, and announces which medicines to give. An interested second-year resident and the senior hunch over the machine, periodically muttering, "Looks idioventricular" or "I think I see P waves," medical labels describing the heart rhythm.

A common question is, "Has anyone gotten a gas? Can we have a gas, please?" This triggers the frenzied thrusting of needles into the patient's thigh in search of the femoral artery and a specimen of arterial blood. This will be sent to the lab for measurement of its oxygen and carbon dioxide levels, the "blood gas." The blood gas helps determine whether the patient, who is intubated and ventilated with a manually squeezed rubber balloon, is getting enough oxygen. After a great deal of stabbing, blood rushes into a syringe. In a patient who had not been breathing for several minutes prior to the code, the normally bright red arterial blood is oxygen-starved and purplish. This, combined with the proximity of the femoral artery and vein, prompts skepticism on the blood's origin. "Looks venous, too dark to be arterial. Do you think it's venous?" Veins normally carry oxygen-depleted blood, and the accidental puncture of the femoral vein might be one explanation for its dark color. The specimen is sent to the lab regardless, and when the results indicate the oxygen content is indeed low, "Must have been venous, all right," is suggested and incites a new round of thigh stabbing and bloodletting.

What is done best at a code is the generation of an enormous amount of garbage. All of the equipment used is packaged as carefully and purposefully as any other product targeted to a specific consumer group, and the wrappers wind up as garbage. In fact, because most medical equipment is "sterile, single use only," most of the products themselves also wind up as garbage. Wrappings are thrown on the floor and on the patient immediately after the removal of their contents. At the conclusion of the code the bed, patient, and floor are covered with assorted trash, paper, bits of plastic, used needles and syringes, and rubber gloves, all strewn amidst pools of blood.

I remember arriving at a code quite a few minutes after its conclusion in the ICU at NYG. Everybody had left the room though no one had yet elected to start the process of cleaning up. The patient was a middle-aged alcoholic man who'd had pneumonia, gotten septic, and crashed. A really close eye must be kept on infected boozers as they can go down the tubes in a matter of hours, even if they're otherwise young and healthy. I've seen young drinkers in the emergency room with a bit of a cough and fever wind up stone cold dead the next day. This particular patient had coded and gotten back a blood pressure and pulse about five times during the course of the late evening and night before he finally crashed for good. He was fat, pale, and lay dead as the proverbial doornail among the rumpled and bloodied sheets of his bed. I could hear the dim wail of his relatives, who stood waiting about twelve or fifteen strong down the hall in NYG's family waiting area, a stale, dim room just like its equivalent over at MH. The code board, a wooden plank placed under the patient to provide a firm base for chest compressions, was wedged halfway beneath him. An intubation tube, wedged into his trachea, hung from his mouth. Several plastic intravenous catheters hung from his arms, those used to gain access to large blood vessels neatly sewed to the skin. The floor was absolutely covered with garbage. The final code had lasted some time and at least ten yards of electrocardiogram paper lay on the floor in a heap, documenting the final history of the electrical activity of the patient's heart. An arm hung off the bed, the fingers in a comfortable semiflexed position. On the bedside table there was a radio still on, playing rock and roll. Perhaps when the man had first coded he'd been listening to the radio and the code team decided it provided pleasant accompaniment to their task. Mick Jagger, his lips shaking and quavering, hooted, "I can't get no . . . No, no, no! Hey, hey, hey! That's what I say!" into the otherwise silent room of the dead man.

Even more memorable was a code I attended that lasted well over an hour. The senior resident had gone through the treatments for virtually every abnormal heart rhythm in the book; the medical student was starting to chafe his hands from chest compressions; all the lines, both large and small, that anyone could dream up to start had been started; gases galore, both venous and arterial, had been whisked off to the lab; and everyone was bored and antsy to get back to their normal work.

The senior looked up to no one in particular and said, "Does anyone have any suggestions?"

From somewhere in the crowd came the real answer, "Yeah, let's have pizza tonight, instead of Chinese."

Clearly, the issue of "coding" a patient is chock-full of

wonderful ethical and emotional dilemmas. It is one of the most painful and denigrating acts a human being can commit against another human being. It is often of little or no clear benefit to the patient. It depersonalizes doctors and nurses. It is costly. Much the same can also be said about other forms of advanced life support. Intubation and the use of a respirator is brutal, painful, and terrifying. The intra-aortic balloon pump is ghastly. Yet, each of these procedures is extremely common, and thousands of people are subjected to them every day.

In my mind, the rightness or wrongness of critical care has little to do with ethics. To me, the most important question is, "What does the patient want?" The decision about treatment lies foremost with the patient himself. If the wishes of the patient are clear, I see no need for ethical and moral hand wringing. Consider the twenty-eight-year-old alcoholic man who bled to death on the wards at NYG. Despite the fact that his death was a foregone conclusion, his doctors respected his desire to be treated as aggressively as possible. I would have done the same. I may have my own ideas about how I would want to be treated in the same situation, or about what I'd want for a relative, but I'd never force those beliefs on someone else.

One way that a patient can make his wishes clear is to write them down on a piece of paper. Having a lawyer affix at least a half-dozen official-looking signatures and stamps to the paper gives it the power of a "living will," and doctors must abide by its instructions. It might read, "In the event that I am gravely ill and unable to make decisions regarding the use of advanced cardiac life support should it become necessary, and should my chances of recovery to a functional status be remote, I hereby declare that such heroic measures not be taken and that I be allowed to pass away in peace." A right-to-lifer could declare, "Pump on my chest until the last spark has long since disappeared, until my body is cold, stiff, and starting to smell." Whatever the preference, a living will makes the decision about "aggressive life support" and so-called code status clear and removes the burden of decision from the doc.

Unfortunately, living wills are few and far between. In fact, I've never seen one. Another way to find out what a patient wants is to simply sit down and ask him. This is clearly a very delicate task and, mostly out of emotional cowardice, one I rarely attempt. Nonetheless, I occasionally do so, gingerly dancing around the subject, broaching it thus, "Mr. Terminally Ill, it's very difficult for me to bring this up, but have you done any thinking at all about what you would like us to do for you in the event you become critically ill?"

The spectrum of answers to this question is very broad. There are those who refuse to accept the possibility of death and fight it tooth and nail to the end, insisting that everything possible be done. Others reconcile themselves as best they can to dying, focus their energy on living life to the fullest until the end, and request only that they be kept comfortable. Again, the issue is not what they decide, but that they make the decision themselves. This is much easier than not understanding what a patient wants and, when it's time to start the real torture, having to make the decision for him.

I should add that not all doctors share this sentiment. A doctor's ethical beliefs about his medical duties can go a long way in directing his actions, even if they go against the patient's wishes. For some, this is purely passive, for example in refusing to perform abortions. In others it is active and emphatic, like refusing to respect a patient's explicit instructions not to be coded.

Unfortunately, most docs do not inquire as to a patient's wishes in the event of his death. It's much easier to just treat the patient and worry about his death when the time comes than to start getting touchy-feely and teary-eyed with everybody right off the bat. Remember, residency is a time to build barriers, not to start baring one's own, or other people's, feelings. Furthermore, most patients do not have a living will. The result is that the vast majority of deaths occur without any clear sense of how the patient wants to be managed. For most, "code status" is a decision made by doctors who may not have the patient's best interests in mind.

A recent flurry of academic research on the human aspects of critical care and advanced life support is beginning to help remedy this situation. Such research, it is hoped, will raise doctors' awareness about the importance of patients' feelings, and encourage them to ask the difficult question, "What do you want us to do for you if you die?" One of the medical journals ran an article a few years ago about the feelings of people who'd survived in-hospital codes. The authors looked up the records of a large number of patients who'd been coded. Of these something on the order of 30 percent survived the code and perhaps 10 percent made it to the point of leaving the hospital. Of this 10 percent, an even smaller fraction had enough of their brains left to reply to the question, "Are you glad you were coded?" Few were, and fewer yet would elect to have it done again. A poor average, which, given the severity of illness in most patients who are coded, should come as little surprise.

After witnessing several hundred codes, some nine years after starting medical school, I met a lady in the emergency room who said she'd died and been brought back by the doctors. I asked her if she was glad they had done so and she smiled and said, "Oh, yes!"

One week later I met a middle-aged man who'd also survived a code. On the night I met him he'd come to the emergency room complaining of chest pain. I planned to admit him to make sure he had not had a heart attack. Since all the beds in the hospital were full, he spent the night sitting on a stretcher in the emergency room. In fact, because there would be no discharges at night, his only hope for getting out of the emergency room and into a bed was that someone on one of the floors would die. He spoke only Spanish so I couldn't quiz him in detail about being coded, but as I worked through the night and glanced in on him, I noted his apparent pleasure to be alive. He spent the night flirting shamelessly with the lady lying on the stretcher next to his.

The issue of coding those who are essentially dead, those who have been in a long downhill slide for weeks or months in the hospital, is also being more closely examined by medical researchers. They have identified groups of patients that virtually never survive more than a few days after a code, provided they make it through the code itself. They argue against coding these patients, claiming that it does not represent good medical care. Put differently, if death is inevitable either way, code or no, the procedure is of no benefit to the patient and need not even be considered as a part of his medical care. I await further data in this field with bated breath.

Although I enjoy knocking docs for failing to include the patient in the code status decision, they are not always wholly to blame. The patient himself often cannot participate in the discussion. This is most common in the elderly, extremely demented, and critically ill patient from a nursing home. These patients arrive in the hospital like so many sacks of flour, and take about as active a part in their own fate. In such cases the doctor is obligated to speak with the patient's closest relatives and ask them what they want done. In my opinion, clearly understanding the desires of the family is the most important part of this kind of patient's medical care. After all, if the patient is so deeply entombed in a dementia as to be totally unaware of his own predicament, the emotional issues of the case rest almost completely with the family. It is they who grieve or rejoice. For the patient, the experience simply continues his sluglike existence, punctuated by a flurry of needle sticks.

In these cases the family's main concern is the patient's quality of life. "What kind of life will he have if he survives?" "Will treating him cause him to suffer?" I try desperately not to let my proeuthanasia bent spill into my tone of voice when I answer these questions, so that the family can decide on the basis of cold, cruel fact. Relatives often dislike this approach and ask for advice on a personal level. "As a human being, knowing what you know as a doctor, what would you choose? Would you want it for one of your own relatives?" My answer is always the same. Were a relative of mine critically ill and severely and irreversibly demented, I would not allow doctors to impose the torture of a code. Period. No need to dance around and hedge and apologize and cover my bets if the patient is one of my own. If life already offers almost nothing, there's no need to add a few horrendously painful hours of life in the ICU. Advanced cardiac life support, baloney. It's torment, plain and simple. For those who are demented I make it clear that the best outcome, should the patient recover physically, is continued, and probably worsened, dementia. Although I do not know if the dead feel pain while being coded I believe the procedure to be extremely undignified. And no, I would certainly not choose it for one of my own, or for myself.

If the family agrees that the patient is not to be coded I state, "You understand this means that if your relative stops breathing we will not attempt to breathe for him artificially, that if his heart stops beating we will not press on his chest to establish an artificial pulse or administer drugs to restart the heart, and if his blood pressure drops very low we will do nothing more than give intravenous fluids to bring it back up again?" It's one of the few times that I am direct and clear with family members. When the answer is yes I document in the patient's chart that these measures were explicitly discussed with the responsible, named family members and, on this basis, that the patient is a "no code."

Of course, not everybody who gets good and sick starts out as a vegetable. I cared for many critically ill patients who'd been normal and functional at home before suddenly starting to die. Still, for those who arrived in the hospital in a coma, the burden of decision again fell to the family. One man described his mother as "eighty-eight going on seventeen." I never pushed toward a no-code decision in such cases because the chances for recovery could change dramatically in the first twenty-four hours. It wasn't possible to know how much of the patient's physiologic and mental function might recover. Many times this uncertainty resulted in intubation and aggressive care despite the lack of a clear decision about code status. For me, intubating and coding this kind of patient was appropriate and just, and I've never had bad feelings about doing so.

One of the worst ethical dilemmas arose in the previously functional patient who was aggressively treated, intubated, coded, and sent to the expensive care unit but failed to regain any of his old spunk. When I was on the wards, I had many formerly awake and alert patients who'd become suddenly ill, wound up in the ICU in a coma, regained little or no brain function after several days (speaking medically we'd say, "The patient, given a trial of several days of aggressive therapy in the intensive care unit, failed to regain significant mental functioning"), and were shipped off to the wards to die and make room for a new crop in the unit.

On receiving such a transfer I was often told, "The bad news is you're getting a transfer, the good news is it's only a TCTD [to Cloud to die]."

These patients were problematic because being already on respirators they had little chance to stop breathing and die, despite being advertised as TCTD. Typically, they suffered infection after infection and could remain on the respirator for years. Hospitals for the chronically ill are packed with patients like these, many of whom have been long since forgotten by all save the nursing staff.

We had an interesting method of evaluating whether such a patient had any functioning squash (brain) remaining at all. Using the respirator, the patient was pumped up furiously, and then the machine turned off. By doing so the relative amounts of both oxygen and carbon dioxide in the patient's blood were changed completely (these gases are

249

virtually the only two of importance in human physiology). By raising the concentration of oxygen delivered by the respirator the oxygen content of the blood was increased to two or three times normal. The concentration of carbon dioxide (a waste product produced by the body in the process of normal metabolism, excreted through the lungs in expired air), on the other hand, was brought way below normal simply by increasing the number of mechanical breaths delivered per minute. Thus, by simply fiddling with the dials on the machine it was possible to saturate a patient with oxygen and almost completely deplete him of carbon dioxide.

When the machine was then turned off, the oxygen in the patient's blood slowly dropped (as that in the blood was used up by the tissues) while carbon dioxide increased (as it was produced by the tissues and released into the blood). After about five minutes, carbon dioxide would rise way above normal, though oxygen still would not have dropped below dangerous values. This maneuver was not risky to a patient so long as the oxygen level was not allowed to drop below normal before the machine was turned back on.

In human beings, a part of the brain called the brain stem uses rising carbon dioxide as a signal to trigger breathing. This action, a so-called primitive, or visceral, function, is evolutionarily ancient. It is controlled much the same way in a lizard as a human. If the patient failed to breathe on his own after accumulating carbon dioxide for five to ten minutes, this was believed to be a fairly good indication of "brain death," that the brain was functionless, that it had closed shop, retired, and headed for Cloud 9.

Formerly walking, talking, but now comatose, patients were evaluated for remaining brain function in this fashion before going TCTD. I'd look in the patient's chart to see that the pertinent big-cheese docs, especially the head of neurology, were clear on a dismal prognosis for recovery of brain function. If this was the case I'd be blunt with the family about the patient's chances for ever walking and talking again.

The family's next question, inevitably, was, "What will happen to my relative now?"

I'd reply, "Well, he'll probably get some kind of infection within a week or so, whether it's pneumonia or a urinary infection or whatever, usually that is what happens to bed-ridden patients on respirators."

"And then what happens?"

"Well, it can be treated with antibiotics or it can be not treated at all."

"What happens if you treat it with antibiotics?"

"Your relative will remain on the respirator and develop another infection in another few weeks."

"And if you don't treat it, then what happens?"

"Then your relative will die of the infection within a few days, a week at most."

"You mean he won't be treated at all?"

"Not exactly. He'll certainly be given IV fluids and Tylenol for fever."

"Will it be painful?"

"I don't know."

"Is he in pain now?"

"I don't know."

"Will it be painful when he dies?"

"I don't know."

It was unusual in situations like this to reach a discussion of code status. Most families of a living-dead, respirator-bound patient opted for "fluids and Tylenol only." These patients uniformly died within ten days, never even getting a temp by virtue of round-the-clock Tylenol doses administered via feeding tube.

Strangely, the most grateful families I ever dealt with were the ones to whom I explained, in this fashion, how their relatives might simply be allowed to die. I'd even get phone calls two or three days after the patient died from a relative who'd say, "I just want to thank you for all you've done for my relative and for all of us."

In fact, all I'd done was allow the family to instruct me to do nothing at all.

I should add that I never, *ever* made the decision not to treat a comatose, respirator-bound patient without explicit instructions from the patient's family. Again, if it's not one of my own, the ethical dilemma is not mine to sort out. Again also, if it is one of my own, the answer to the ethical dilemma is very clear.

Both right-to-lifers and radical lefties, proverbially strange bedfellows, have honed righteous arguments against euthanasia. Their reasons are widely divergent, but each objects to the concept fundamental to euthanasia, that there is such a thing as a life not worth living.

Right-to-lifers, pounding the Bible, claim all life is sacred and declare that euthanasia is murder, plain and simple. The same argument backs their views on abortion, though one may find among them an oddly favorable attitude toward the death penalty. Lefties fear that accepting the concept that some human life is not worth living will usher in an era of precedented social pathology, the precedents being Nazi experimentation and genocide, the Tuskegee experiments (for those who are unaware of this illuminating example of medical research, the Tuskegee experiments involved the intentional withholding by physicians of treatment from rural black men suffering from syphilis, and the observation, over a period of decades, of the natural course of the disease), or any other historic example of societally sanctioned human abuse. To the lefty, allowing a critically ill, severely demented patient to die is soon followed by the wholesale slaughter of the old, the lame, and the poor.

To both the left and the right I have only one defense for my views. As honorable a pursuit as the preservation of life is for 99 percent of people, there is the 1 percent for whom it is torment. To me the problem is not an ethical dilemma regarding the sanctity of life, or victimizing those for whom there are no advocates, but regret at keeping someone alive with methods that amount to almost constant torture. For the ethicist who needn't carry out orders and relentlessly abuse the patient, it is easy to say a life must be preserved despite the cost in human anguish. As far as I'm concerned, the left- or right-wing moralist is welcome to come into the hospital and stab the patient seven to ten times a day for blood, shove a tube into his penis for a specimen of urine, into his nose for a gob of infected snot, into his stomach for feeding, and into his mouth to unclog a blocked airway. The moralist can, without the patient's or the family's specific written or verbal consent, irradiate the patient daily for chest X rays, poke him twice or thrice a day to replace his IV and, when the patient codes, break his ribs doing chest compressions, shove a tube into his trachea, and bayonet his thighs for arterial blood. In fact, if he wants, he can cut the patient's chest open and manually squeeze the heart to maintain a pulse. All of this, I'm sure, will be done gladly and cheerfully, with the moral righteousness of knowing a life is worth saving at all costs.

For me, one of the lessons of internship and residency was that the preservation of life at all costs did not necessarily fulfill my lifelong wish to be "of service to my fellow man." To me, there were those for whom modern medicine and technology was a clear disservice. For these very few I have become tired of delivering this kind of "health care" and support the concept that among this small minority of patients, the critically ill who have lost the cerebral functions that once made them human, death is preferable to endless torture.

Despite being a nearly endless source for noble and high-sounding philosophizing, the decision to treat or not to treat, to code or not to code, is nearly always based on the more practical consideration of legal responsibility. Lawyers lurk in every medical-ethical nook and cranny. In reality we all fear that in today's highly litigious environment the decision not to code will result in a lawsuit. Therefore, opting to code is much easier than opting not to. A doc may believe in his heart that not coding is in the best interests of the patient, but it is certainly not in his own best interests. In the end we code many people more for our own health than for that of the patient. We simply torment the dead body for a half hour, and eliminate the chance of winding up on the witness stand sputtering and drooling when the attorney for the patient's family asks, "So tell us, Doctor, tell us exactly why you elected not to attempt to restore breath and life to the now deceased husband of poor widow Jones. Can you do that, Doctor?" The first rule of medicine, remember, is "CYA," "cover your ass."

Being stuck between salivating lawyers on the one side and the all but dead on the other has led to a number of variations on the full-fledged code, the "show code" and the "slow code." These procedures are designed specifically to ensure that, on the one hand, the patient is allowed to die, while on the other, no lawyer gets rich.

I did a "show code" on a man with AIDS when I was a supervising resident on the wards at NYG. The patient was a young junkie, about twenty-two years old, riddled with mycobacterium avian-intracellulare, or MAI. MAI is a variant of mycobacterium tuberculosis, the bug that causes TB. AIDS patients get both TB and MAI. The patient had been on every anti-TB drug known to man and though the bugs were still frolicking about in most of his internal organs (everywhere the consulting docs stuck a needle they found MAI) he was fairly stable and, one day, we discharged him with instructions to keep taking the drugs at home.

He came back two days later looking absolutely terrible, probably because he hadn't been correctly taking his forty daily pills. My team was on long call and we readmitted him to the hospital on a terribly busy night. The intern assigned to work up the patient was trapped somewhere in a miasma of clogged IVs so I decided to give him a break and deal with the patient until he had the time. I did a history and physical and called the bug specialist to discuss antibiotics. I sat at the nurses' station and wrote out the list of med orders and stopped back in the patient's room to tell him what we'd be doing for him.

He was terribly short of breath and anxious and kept asking for something to calm down. I initially refused to give him any kind of sedative, fearing even the mildest would depress his respirations and calm him down for good. Nonetheless, he was so frightened that I finally relented, giving him a homeopathic dose of Valium.

I returned to the nurses' station and called the X-ray tech to come up and take an X ray of the patient's chest. The tech went into his room while I was sitting at the nurses' station. I watched her walk by, the lumbering X-ray machine beeping along at a half mile an hour in front of her.

After about two minutes she came walking out of the room and said, "Uh, are you the doctor for this patient?"

I said, "Yes," and she said, "I think you should come and have a look at him, I think he's passed away."

I jogged into the room with a few of the nurses and, sure enough, the patient was dead. Not stone cold dead, but fresh dead, with a burning cigarette hanging from his hand, which lay draped off the edge of the bed.

I sighed and looked at the nurses. "He's dead and I really don't think we should code him. It would just be an insult because he isn't going to make it and if he does he won't last for long."

They nodded because they agreed, but we were all clearly nervous about this decision. An image of a silk-suited lawyer smugly addressing me on the witness stand flashed through my mind. I said, "The hell with it. Call a code."

The nurses nodded again and went off to have the operator announce the code on the PA system. I heard, "CAC Nine North! CAC Nine North!" while I was intubating the patient. One of the nurses did chest compressions until the team arrived. My intern came flying into the room and, when he saw that it was his patient who'd coded, realized he'd been saved hours of work and broke into a tremendous grin.

When I saw this I told him, "You're filling out the death certificate *and* calling the family to inform them *and* getting consent from them for the autopsy," and he stopped grinning. We pumped on the patient's chest for about ten minutes, gave him the routine cardiac meds, and drew a few blood gases, which were uniformly awful. When we reached the point where we could say we had done everything, I called (ended) the code. I spent the next few days convinced that the Valium had killed the patient and feeling relieved that we'd done a "show code," a code performed so anyone concerned could be shown the record indicating that the patient was coded when he died.

A slow code is a variation on a show code. A slow code is done on a patient who everyone knows is going to die, but for whom there are explicit code instructions. When the patient finally kicks, everybody wanders over and codes him in a sort of desultory, halfhearted way, waiting enough time so the patient can be declared finally and everlastingly dead, dead, dead.

It has become legal in the last year or two to document a patient's code status and, although this requires the completion of a six-page form, this is a definite step forward. By allowing a doc to create a signed record of the patient's or family's wishes, it is helping make codes performed for fear of litigation, rather than for the patient's best interests, a thing of the past.

15

Kids

I waded and complained and battled my way through the internship year and, for the grand finale, was tossed onto the pediatrics wards for the final few months. I'm tempted to say that the bullshit and feelings and emotions and craziness and screwups and the rest of it were all the same in peds as in adults except that the patients were smaller, but that isn't really how I felt. The kids were divided among the majority who had acute problems that could get fixed quickly, the minority who were sick with chronic illnesses, and the few who were sick as dogs and either died quickly or wasted away for a few years and then died no matter what you did. Dealing with sick-as-dogs kids had a harder edge for me than dealing with sick-as-dogs adults, their being just kids and all, but that probably only means that I didn't spend enough time in peds to get really good and hard and cynical about children.

Most people make a lot of noise about the inherent resiliency and natural tendency toward healing and normalcy possessed by children. My experience in peds demonstrated that for the most part this was true. I remember my amazement in watching children almost desperately shake rattles or scrutinize toys while being poked and prodded by doctors. Such children seemed naturally driven toward health and vigor. Nonetheless, many, many kids got critically ill and did their best to die in a manner even the sickest adult would envy.

Most of my experience on the peds wards was spent doing what pediatricians called "bread and butter" pediatrics, illnesses comprising the vast majority of admissions among different age groups. On the infants' ward, for example, bread-and-butter peds consisted of treating asthma, D and D (diarrhea and dehydration), FIBs ("fever in babies"), pneumonia, fractures, and sundry other conditions. These were kids in need only of a little help to get better, doing most of the healing on their own. They were the strong, resilient ones who insisted on living normal kid lives despite being in the hospital.

Asthmatic babies (ped interns' slang, "wheezlers") lived in "mist tents," big, clear plastic hoods placed over their cribs and pumped full of thick cool mist by vaporizers. Walking into a wheezler's room revealed a fog-filled tent; looking really carefully into the mist might allow a glimpse of a hazy kid busily sucking on his toes or babbling to himself and shaking a rattle as though nothing at all unusual was happening. We'd unzip the tents once or twice a day and stick our stethoscopes onto the kids to see if they were wheezing. After a few days they'd stop and we'd send them home.

D and D's were almost always babies. Having had a bad case of diarrhea, they'd shit themselves a little bit too much and get dehydrated. Seen in the emergency room they looked like miniature Mr. Krams, pruned up with dry skin and little, pinched, wizened faces. The anterior fontanelle (the funny soft spot young babies have just above the forehead, formed because the skull bones have not yet quite met) would be slightly sucked in because even their pint-sized brains were low on water. D and D's were admitted and poked with IVs for "rehydration." After getting about half a liter of fluid, they'd fill out like a dry sponge being soaked with water and become their laughing, gurgling, whining, toe-sucking selves again within a day or two.

FIBs were babies under the age of two months who had a fever. Pediatricians, having decided that there was no way to tell if an under-two-month-old was sick just by looking at it, admitted and treated all young babies with fever. I say "just by looking at it" because your normal older kid tends to look sick when ill: cranky, irritable, refusing to eat or sleep, and being a big pain in the ass. The sick under-two-month-old is often unable to make enough of a ruckus to be a pain in the ass. A healthy baby, hungry and neglected for a little while, raises a shriek that is almost unbelievable given its size. An unhealthy one might only be able to raise a pathetic whimper. The only clue to a life-threatening infection in such a baby may be fever and a slightly gorky appearance.

I hated FIBs because the big-time infection work-up was brutal and, nine times out of ten, came back negative, meaning the kid probably had a virus and didn't need to be treated at all. Since there was no way to know this beforehand, we were obligated to torture and treat every FIB just to be sure.

"Just to be sure" was as big a catch phrase in peds as in adult medicine. It's just another way of saying "CYA." Possibly the greatest medical nightmare in terms of potential for a lawsuit was sending a kid with a fever ("febrile child") home and learning a week later that he was admitted the following day to another hospital with meningitis and permanent neurologic damage. This was worse, financially speaking, than the child dying, because the malpractice suit would seek compensation and support payments for *the rest of the child's life*.

The FIB work-up on a child about a foot and a half

long was horrible. He'd have a lumbar puncture (LP), chest X ray, around twenty needle sticks for various blood tests, urine cultures (often obtained via the truly ghastly "suprapubic tap," in which a needle was stuck right through the kid's abdominal wall into his bladder), multiple stabs to place an IV, and admission to the hospital for both intravenous and intramuscular antibiotics until the fever resolved and the blood tests came back normal. A ten-pound babe was easily stuck thirty times in a three-day stay. The LP was absolutely vicious. A coworker grabbed the child by the neck and rear end and bent him in half, and the doc stuck a needle into the base of his spine until the clear fluid came dripping out. The process of folding the kid in half was fondly known as "bending the child like a chicken."

One of the blood tests we did on FIBs was a blood culture. This was to make sure that the source of the kid's fever wasn't a blood-borne infection. Every once in a while a blood culture came back positive, generating extraordinary excitement among the pediatricians. Endless discussions ensued about whether the cultured bacterium might be a contaminant resulting from putting the needle through inadequately cleaned skin, or perhaps because the specimen was handled by a grubby intern. Other topics of heated dissension included how long the child would need to stay in the hospital, whether to treat the infection (if real) with oral or intravenous antibiotics, and the rest of it. The old-timer docs who'd been around since before penicillin mumbled about how these infections probably didn't even require treatment, that they were transient and happened in every normal kid at one time or another. They believed there were a hundred such infections happening in people's homes for every one we were seeing in the hospital, and that these children were doing just fine without being tormented by doctors. Through all of this the kid would be in his crib sucking on his toes or babbling or crying, trying to live a normal life despite being in the hospital.

The vast majority of kids with run-of-the-mill problems on the general peds ward got better mostly by themselves. They were the strong, self-healing, resilient types. Despite this we kept our brows continually furrowed waiting for the kid who was going to crash, the one who wouldn't look so bad and then suddenly box. It was this fear that motivated many a pediatric admission. There was a sense that although children were resilient and all that jazz, they had a fairly small margin from which they could bounce back. Pushed just a bit too far they would crash fast. This fear, it seemed to me, kept the kid docs in a constant state of ulcerogenic anxiety that made them push and medicate and work up the kids relentlessly.

The fact of the matter was that they were right. Inevitably, an okay-looking kid turned out to have an "overwhelming" problem, like a whopping case of meningitis, got overwhelmed by it, and waddled up to Cloud 9 to meet his great-grandparents; but this was rare.

Most of the kids on the infants' ward had acute, sudden-onset, short-term illness like diarrhea and dehydration or fever. As strange as it seems there were also kids, babies, who were chronically ill. This was especially the case among kids with bizarre heart defects, whom we called "cardiacs," and those with severe lung problems. At any given time there were one or two kids with bronchopulmonary dysplasia, or BPD, on the infants' ward. Although these kids should logically have been referred to as "lungers," I've heard that phrase used only in reference to adults.

Most of the BPD kids had been born too early and spent long periods in the neonatal ICU because of their underdeveloped lungs. They'd spent so much time on respirators—weeks, or even months—and had so many infections that their lungs had become twisted and scarred.

They'd be discharged after protracted ICU stays, but were continually readmitted when their chests got congested and infected at home. In the hospital, we'd give them antibiotics and put them in mist tents, where they'd wheeze and cough and sputter until they got better.

Watching the nurses give chest therapy to the BPD and asthma kids was one of the few heartwarming sights in the hospital. A nurse would lay a kid facedown on her lap, with his head hanging between her knees and, with classically sure hands, pound on his back like she was playing a little squirming human bongo drum. Although they'd get pounded pretty fiercely the kids seemed to like it, and quietly allowed themselves to be beat up. The pounding loosened up all the junk and crap down in the their lungs ("secretions"), and helped them cough it up. I'd wander onto the ward late at night and discover a row of nurses sitting at the nurses' station, gabbing and gossiping and pounding on these blissed-out kids, who lay draped in their laps. It really was heartwarming.

The BPD kids, being chronically sick, were regulars on the ward and well known to the nurses, who behaved just like mothers, cuddling and scolding them. Each spent about a week at home after leaving the hospital before having to come back for another month of antibiotics, mist, and pounding.

In spite of my earlier lip service about a vague, poorly defined sympathy for children, the reality for those on the peds housestaff was little different from the reality of those on the adult medicine ward. The first rule was "CYA" and the second, do whatever is necessary to get the hell out of the hospital. Again, this was more the result of the system of training, the fact that the housestaff was continually being browbeaten, than because there was anything inherently wrong with them as people. An intern might start peds with some sense that children are innocent, beautiful, and graceful, but after a few horrendous nights on call, all of that crap was blown clean away and the beautiful little kids became patients. The previously alluded to sense of sympathy that found kids little and cute didn't have much bearing in the heat of battle. What had to be done had to be done regardless of how un-nice it was.

In fact, because the kids really were so blessed cute most of the procedures done on them seemed crueler than their equivalents in adults; thus an even harder exterior was necessary to shield oneself from one's actions.

The kiddies did not sit still when they were subject to medical torture. Adults often cooperated when told not to move if they didn't want to go through the same procedure all over again. Such undisguised threats did not work with children. If a procedure was genuinely painful a kid screamed his little head off until it stopped. The only way to avoid this was to sedate the child, but this could not be done every time you needed to stick one for blood.

I was struck by the singularity of purpose in children screaming from torment. Babies undergoing FIB torture put their entire bodies into the expression of their anguish. I've seen babies shriek, squirm, puff up, turn completely red, and produce impossible quantities of snot and tears for hours, all the while being mercilessly stuck and called "little shits." It seemed the equivalent of an adult exerting himself fully and totally for the same period. Even a marathon runner doesn't work himself as fully as a child screaming during a FIB work-up.

In the United States, sick children have classes of illness related to both age and socioeconomic class. The causes of morbidity and mortality among neonates (in plain English, causes of sickness and death in newborn babies), for example, differ widely between the rich and the poor. In an affluent community the problems faced by neonates are mostly so-called obstetrical events or congenital defects. An

263

"obstetrical event" means that everything is going along just fine until an unforeseen problem develops during labor that causes trouble for mom or baby. For example, a kid is born feet first instead of head first, or chokes on his own umbilical cord. A congenital defect means the kid is put together wrong (a common question after delivery relates to this: "Does the baby have ten fingers and ten toes?") and develops related problems. Life-threatening congenital defects often involve the heart being built wrong and pumping blood in the wrong direction to the wrong places.

Considering poorer people, the problems of newborns are more often infectious, or related to low birth weight and premature birth. A "low birth weight" baby is one who is born too small, and a premature baby one who is born too early (premies are usually too small, as well). That these problems account for the majority of illnesses suffered by infants of poor people doesn't mean they don't also suffer the ailments found in their wealthier counterparts. Thus, poor people have a higher infant mortality rate than rich people. Surprise, surprise.

The "infant mortality rate" measures how many babies per thousand live births die up to a given age. Though the United States prides itself on having a very low IMR (around the twelfth- or thirteenth-lowest in the world at approximately 10 deaths per 1,000 births), drastically large differences are found between the rich and poor. Rich white folks have a rate down around 8 per 1,000, while poor black folks are losing 20 or 25 of every 1,000 children they deliver. In general, when a poor person obtains a good place to live, decent food to eat, a good education, adequate prenatal care, and all the other stuff that liberals like to scream about, their babies do much better.

As babies get a bit older (up to around six months) they get more robust. Still, the "socioeconomic" differences in cause of illness persist. In general there aren't a whole lot of hospitalized rich six-month-olds, and a high proportion suffer unavoidable problems, like elective surgery for cleft lips and palates, undescended testicles, and the occasional need for some kind of intestinal or cardiac surgery. Poorer babies still tend to get infections like pneumonia and meningitis, in addition to having elective surgical and less acute medical needs.

After about a year and a half to two years kids are thought of in terms of their medical problems as children. While short-term, acute illness is the norm among babies, the age group between late infancy and adolescence sees more long-term or chronic disease. In psychological and social development there is constant change, a newborn becomes an infant, an older baby, a toddler, a young child, an older child, and an adolescent. The social differences in causes for admission persist. In wealthier kids, you see probably less child abuse, trauma, and infections than among poor kids. I hedge and say "probably less child abuse" because a major gap may exist in the amount of child abuse that occurs versus that actually reported among richer folks. Better-off middle-aged kids (say five to ten years) tend to be admitted for horrendous things like cancer, esoteric diseases like juvenile arthritis and bizarre forms of anemia, "bread and butter" chronic illnesses like asthma and diabetes, or quick-fix problems like fractures and minor trauma. Poorer kids also suffer these problems, and are the victims of more (reported) violence, big-time trauma, and infectious disease.

The children's ward, which housed kids two to thirteen or fourteen years old, had the highest proportion of dying kids. Cancer, especially leukemia, strikes more kids than people realize or like to believe. The children's ward at MH always had several kids with leukemia and it always felt like the proportion of kids with cancer to self-healing types was very high.

Cancer and the threat of death in a child was a very big

deal. While your average old person with cancer might not elicit a whole lot of attention and sympathy ("Well, at least he had a long and full life," etc.), cancer in a child was always a matter for very serious and hushed tones.

Every cancer kid at MH had a private doc who headed a very intense team approach to his case. In the hierarchy the pediatric housestaff didn't rate very high. Having a kid with cancer as a patient usually meant sitting in silence at yet another very serious conference, and doing a tremendous amount of scut work on the patient. The intern drew the blood, stuck in the line, and stood back while the ped onc doc came along and torched the child with chemotherapy. A tense period followed during which the intern tortured the patient ceaselessly to determine if the drugs would work before the side effects killed him.

When I was on the wards the basic premise in treating leukemia, cancer of the white blood cells, was essentially the same as that in treating cancer in adults like the Lady with Lung Cancer, and poor, deluded, ice-cream-craving Mr. Smith. It went, "Kill rapidly dividing cells!"

In leukemia, the specific target of the drugs was the bone marrow, the producer of white blood cells. The bone marrow was full of what the blood docs called stem cells, which matured into full-grown white cells. The chemotherapy killed stem cells, whether healthy or cancerous. The goal of treatment, more specifically, was, "Destroy every last immature white blood cell in the child's body, healthy and cancerous, and pray that the new set that grows back does not also have cancer." Interestingly, the goal of destroying bone marrow in leukemia was a regrettable side effect in other cancers, one that left the patient vulnerable to infection because of the lack of white cells.

I imagined that the cancer drugs ravaged and burned the bone marrow, like commandos on a search-and-destroy mission, or the atom bomb incinerating Hiroshima. After the treatment was finished the oncologist came along and stabbed the kid in the behind with a gigantic needle and removed a cylindrical chunk of bone marrow from his pelvis, sort of like a petroleum company engineer boring core samples from deep in the earth to look for oil. The specimen was then sliced into incredibly thin sections, stained with red and blue dyes, and examined under the microscope for signs of life. The image in my mind depicted the bone marrow as scorched and blackened, an occasional stunned white blood cell wandering around with third-degree burns. In actuality, all the onc doc would see was big holes in the places that, before treatment, were filled with busily dividing normal and cancerous cells.

After a child received his drugs, there was a brief lag period before the shit hit the fan. After a few hours, suffering the combined emetic effect on the brain and toxic effect on the intestines, the child began to vomit. Sometimes antivomiting ("antiemetic") drugs helped ease the vomiting and sometimes not. Medical jargon for the latter is "intractable vomiting." Marijuana, believed by many to be the best antiemetic agent for chemotherapy patients, is now commercially available in pill form for this use.

Several days of fingernail chewing followed while we waited for the kid to spike a temperature and develop pneumonia from his lack of white blood cells. I'd go into each cancer kid's room at seven every morning and stab him for blood. A normal white blood count (remember, that's the number of white cells in a given volume of blood) is about 5,000-8,000. The leukemia kids started out with astronomically high white counts from all the cancerous cells floating around in their veins, like in the hundreds of thousands, and then, after the medication, dropped down to 1,000, 500, 250, and even down under 50.

We'd say, "Well, it looks like the kiddie has bottomed out his white count," as though it were the kid himself who was responsible for his predicament.

At this point a child could get pneumonia and die from watching someone sneeze on television. Everyone who went in his room wore a gown, cap, and mask to protect the child from getting germs. We called this reverse isolation. Naturally, the nicer the kid, the more likely he was to develop a fever, which obligated a complete fever work-up, including chest X rays, blood cultures, sputum cultures (getting kids to cough voluntarily was difficult, making them breathe mist through a face mask sometimes helped), urine cultures, and lumbar punctures. Then he'd be given bizarre antibiotics to treat the bizarre infections that may have developed.

In the very best of circumstances, the fever and pneumonia were cured or never developed, and a new batch of normal, noncancerous white blood cells grew back. The kid was then sent home. In cancer lingo this first round of treatment was called "induction." The child had to come back to the cancer clinic to have his blood rechecked about every few weeks, and every several months was readmitted and retorched with a minichemotherapy treatment just to make sure. The pediatric cancer docs found that kids who didn't get the "just to make sure" blast of drugs were more likely to relapse with cancer than those who did. This extra blast was called "maintenance." There was also "amplification," though I don't know what it was, and if the cancer stayed away the child was said to be in remission. If the cancer failed to recur after a set number of years he was cured.

The amazing thing about all of this was that given certain kinds of leukemia and certain kinds of patients, it often worked. Twenty years ago kids who got leukemia died, period.

As I remember it, acute lymphocytic leukemia was the best kind for a kid to get if he wanted to live. There were dozens of different additional criteria whose presence altered a child's statistical odds of making it. Such criteria

268

related to the particular kind of acute lymphocytic leukemia afflicting the child, age, whether the child was a he or
a she, and so on.

A type of leukemia called acute myelogenous leukemia
had a particularly dismal prognosis. Most of the kids who
were treated for it went into remission but relapsed
quickly. They'd be readmitted for "reinduction," though
everyone knew the chances for survival were dismal.

I did the scut on a kid who was being treated for his
fourth relapse of AML. Everyone knew he was going to
die and had leveled with his parents about it. They refused
to accept this and insisted he be treated and treated and
treated. He was about half the normal size for a child his
age because of all the weight he'd lost and the growing he'd
been unable to do, and hadn't had a hair on his head for
several months. He cried every time he saw anyone with a
stethoscope. I'm certain he is dead today.

One of the other kinds of cancer kids tend to get is a
bone tumor called osteogenic sarcoma. As I remember it,
this tumor formed in the bone, destroyed it, and metasta-
sized to other organs. The only way to cure it was by
chopping it out before it had a chance to spread.

I saw two cases, both in kids who were on the children's
ward when I worked there. Both kids had the tumor in the
femur (thigh) bone, which, I dimly remember, was a common place for it to make its first appearance. Right up
until just before I started working on the ward, OS of the
femur was treated simply by cutting the kid's leg off above
the tumor (an above-the-knee amputation, or AKA), a
procedure, as you might imagine, that put quite a crimp
in a kid's life-style.

A friend of mine, a physical therapist who helps physically disabled people learn to overcome their disabilities,
considers the knee to be the most important organ below
the rib cage. Admittedly, this is a slightly extreme reflection of her physical therapy bias, but she does have a

point. An intact set of knees allows a person to walk, run, jump, squat, kick, dance, leap, dash, saunter, hop, skip, tap, and all the other things a person normally does with his legs. If a person's knees are missing or busted these activities can still be attempted, but never as well as when they were intact.

My friend told me that were she forced to choose an injury involving an amputation of some significant part of her body it would never be an AKA, but a BKA, a below-the-knee amputation. Granted that feet are important, she'd explain, but not nearly as important as knees. She said she'd trained countless people with BKAs to lead completely normal lives. Given enough time, care, a good prosthesis, and an intact set of knees, they could do all the things they'd been able to do before the amputation. AKAs, on the other hand, went through long, difficult periods of learning to cope with knee prostheses and never reached a level of proficiency as close to normal as the BKAs.

Imagine, then, that a school-aged kid develops a funny pain in the thigh. Mommy whisks her babe to the doctor and wham bang two weeks later he's falling on his face in a hospital ward trying to learn to use his new wooden leg with its trick knee. Having recognized the horribleness of this prospect, some creative pediatric orthopedists (kid bone docs) came up with a terrific, radical new way to minimize the trauma of OS surgery in kids. They agreed that although the matter was horrible all around, the roughest part for a kid was the loss of his knee. They'd do thousands of OS kids a year a big favor if they figured out a way to preserve their knees.

They came up with a new kind of surgery in which the child had the tumor chopped *out* of his leg, rather than having the entire leg amputated. After cutting the leg off at the upper thigh, above the tumor, the surgeons also severed the leg just below the knee joint. The midportion of the leg, including the knee joint and the tumor, wound up in the garbage. The lower leg, with the foot attached, was turned around backward, and sewn onto the stump of the thigh, with the muscles and ligaments reattached. I know this sounds ridiculous, but this procedure created a knee joint from the backward foot and ankle. The tough bottom surface of the foot, angled so that it faced down and forward, fit neat and cosy into a lower-leg prosthesis. Wagging the ankle mimicked the action of the knee.

I went into the room with the two kids who'd had the surgery and asked if I could look.

They said, "Sure!" whipped back their blankets, and there were two feet glued on backward to two thighs.

I said, "Can you move them around?"

They said, "Sure!" and started waving their feet at each other and laughing. It was bizarre, amazing, and delightful all at the same time.

I said, "Can you move your toes?"

They said, "Sure!" and proceeded to stir up a breeze with ten combined toes.

Only one of the kids had started to learn to use a prosthesis. The kids were in the same room intentionally, one ahead of the other in treatment and therapy. This allowed the second kid to learn and take heart in the experiences of the first. If a fresh OS kid happened along he'd be put in with the second one, and so on until the supply of OS patients ran out. This system of learning, teaching, and supporting worked so well one hoped for a continual staggered stream of kids with bone cancer.

I said to the first kid, "If you don't mind I'd really like to see you use your prosthesis."

He said, "Sure!" whipped on his specially designed artificial lower leg, and marched around the room with it. He barely had a limp.

I spent the very last month of my internship year on the infants' ward, and one of my very last patients as an intern was a terrific baby, a tiny nine-month-old fellow with a heart defect. He was a charming little guy and had a crappy little heart, which, I suppose, is the pediatric confirmation of the "conservation of malignancy theory."

Little babies can develop the bizarrest of heart anatomies while growing in the womb; virtually all of them get into trouble because their hearts do not pump blood correctly. By way of review, remember that the heart contains two separate pumping systems. The right side of the heart, comprised of the right atrium, right ventricle, and the pulmonary artery, delivers oxygen-starved blood to the lungs. The left side of the heart, comprised of the left atrium, left ventricle, and aorta, delivers the freshly oxygenated blood to the body's tissues. All sorts of grotesque derangements can occur in this two-pump system. In one such condition, majestically christened "transposition of the great arteries," the two systems are closed. One endlessly circles blood to and from the lungs, and the other ignominiously shunts choked red corpuscles to the body. Because the two systems do not communicate, the blood cycled to the lungs is never able to release its load of oxygen, while that delivered to the asphyxiated tissues merely gets bluer and bluer.

A baby born with two closed internal circuits that are unable to communicate with each other gets in trouble very quickly when it comes time to breathe. The trouble begins when the baby is born because babies have no need to breathe while inside mommy. An unborn baby floats around in a big bag full of fluid, like in those pictures you used to see in *Life* magazine, and freeloads oxygen from mommy's blood. A big, ugly, dark, reddish-purple organ that looks like a big, wet fungus covered with veins is plastered up against the wall of the womb and, like a true parasite, sucks food and oxygen out of mommy's blood. It is the placenta.

As the baby floats around in the amniotic sac freeloading air from mommy, its fluid-filled, developing lungs do no breathing. Nature, which understands the quiescent nature of fetal lungs, has developed two ingenious methods to divert blood to more needy areas, secret side doors and back exits that almost completely bypass the lungs.

One such secret exit is the truncus arteriosus, a small, unassuming tube that leads blood from the pulmonary artery to the aorta. The pulmonary artery is the blood vessel that normally carries blood from the right side of the heart to the lungs. The aorta, remember, normally carries freshly oxygenated blood from the left side of the heart to the body. Therefore, when blood passes from the pulmonary artery to the truncus, and then to the aorta, it bypasses the lungs altogether. A small amount does manage to seep along the regular tubes to the developing lungs, because, after all, they need a bit of oxygen and food to grow just like the rest of the body.

In the heart itself there is a second side door, a small oval hole covered with a flap. It is located in the right atrium, the chamber that receives blood after its trip to the body. Normally, the right atrium passes blood along to the right ventricle to be sent to the lungs. When the fetal right atrium contracts, a small volume of blood passes through the hole directly to the left atrium. From the left atrium, the blood passes to the left ventricle and back out the aorta, again bypassing the lungs. This system is so simple and graceful that doctors have been forced to give the oval hole a Latin name. Simplicity might force them to lower their fees. The hole has been entitled "foramen ovale," Latin for "oval hole." The entire system of rerouted blood is known as the fetal circulation.

In sum, while the baby is snug and safe inside of mommy, getting all the oxygen it needs from the placenta, it needn't worry about breathing. God and nature have designed the developing heart in a way that allows blood to bypass the lungs, sending almost all of it directly to the developing body. At the moment of birth, however, the baby is cut off from mommy and absolutely must find a new source of oxygen. It must learn to breathe, and fast. The world is a cold, cruel place.

As the baby is squeezed from the womb, most of the fluid in its lungs is also squeezed out. The infant pops out into reality, emits a shriek, and fills its lungs with air. Suddenly, all the doors and side exits that served to divert blood from the lungs receive a magic signal and slam shut. The flap in the foramen ovale plasters itself closed so that blood can no longer escape directly from the right atrium to the left. Blood entering the pulmonary artery finds the ductus arteriosus shut and locked tight, never to open again. Sixty or seventy years later, when the baby goes to the hospital for coronary artery bypass surgery after his first heart attack, the surgeon will point at a hairlike strand of tissue attached to the pulmonary artery and say, "That's the remnant of the ductus arteriosus."

The blood, now diverted to the lungs in the fashion it will follow for the rest of the baby's life, encounters air from his first breath. As planned from the beginning of time, the blood performs its duty of removing oxygen from the air, returns to the left side of the heart, and continues on the first of literally hundreds of millions of such circuits it will make in the baby's lifetime.

With the successful completion of this process, babies go from a dismal and unsettling shade of gray to bright pink in a matter of minutes. Even babies of ethnic groups having a very dark skin color come out gray and pink up once they've figured out how to breathe. A baby who develops breathing or circulatory problems at birth stays this horrible ashen color and may even turn a really fearsome shade of blue. When this happens you don't have to be a doctor to understand that it means trouble, trouble, trouble.

Probably the most traumatic event a human being must

ever endure is being born. Birth is rough for mommy but rougher, I think, for the baby, who goes from a peaceful existence floating in warm fluid, dreaming of nothingness, to being relentlessly pushed into a room somewhere and having to learn to breathe in a period of about thirty seconds. It is a time when God and nature take over two bodies completely. To mommy they say, "Your whole body will be consumed in bringing a new life into the world, you will become a straining, sweating biologic entity over which you will have very little control," and to the new life they say, "Live!! Breathe!!" For those who believe in God it's one of the processes in the world that reaffirms their belief, and for those who believe in nature and evolution it demonstrates forcefully and graphically that the baby has careened into the world after billions and billions of years of change, development, other life, and death.

Clearly, a system as complex and delicate as that of learning to breathe and properly circulate blood is one that can go wrong in many ways. In premature birth the main problem usually relates to lungs that are not yet developed enough to perform their breathing duties. Premature babies may spend long periods breathing supplemental oxygen, or even intubated and attached to mechanical respirators.

In "transposition of the great arteries" (or TPA), as I've explained, the circuits to the lungs and heart are unconnected. This causes no problem in the uterus because oxygen is supplied by mommy, but causes great trouble at birth when the lungs must take over the job of supplying the whole body with oxygen.

Strangely, both the ductus arteriosus and foramen ovale can be of great use in TPA. If they stay open after birth they may allow some of the blood from the closed circuit to the lungs to escape into the closed circuit to the body. Such mixing of blood from the two circuits might provide the body with the minimal amount of oxygen necessary to sur-

275

vive. Perhaps God and nature sometimes know to say, "Don't close!!" when a baby is born with this condition. At times this can buy a baby enough time to be taken to the operating room to have his great vessels rearranged by a pediatric cardiothoracic surgeon (I have a great deal of respect for peds chest surgeons, especially the fact that they've survived something like twelve years of postgraduate training).

On the other hand, if a baby is born with TPA and the ductus and foramen do close, there can be no mixing of blood from the two circuits, no delivery of oxygen to the body, and the baby goes from unsettling ashen gray to horrifying dark blue in less than two minutes. In medical lingo this dark blue oxygenless look is called cyanosis and such heart disease is called cyanotic heart disease. In the former case, the baby gets just enough oxygen to keep from turning blue and is said to have "noncyanotic heart disease."

For the sake of completeness, it should be noted that among babies who are born with normal heart anatomies, trouble occurs if the side doors and back exits *don't* close at birth. When this happens blood continues to be diverted from the lungs at a time when it must go there for oxygen. Varying volumes of blood do manage to reach the lungs along the regular tubes, and afflicted babies turn varying shades of blue. When both the ductus and truncus remain open the baby is said to have "patent ductus arteriosus" and "patent foramen ovale." "Patent" is merely Latin for "Open."

Clearly, cyanotic heart disease is the most life-threatening form of heart disease in children. Kids who are born and stay blue despite being given lots and lots of supplemental oxygen are zoomed off to the "cath lab," where a catheter is shoved into an artery, dye is released, and nifty X-ray movies are taken that demonstrate the heart's anatomy. Sometimes the kids have to get operated on right away if they are to live. Rough way to spend your first day of life. Naturally, the child may die nonetheless. If a child has noncyanotic or only slightly cyanotic heart disease there is more time to sit down, have a cup of coffee, relax a little, and investigate things in a calm manner rather than rushing off to the operating room like a madman.

Again, if a child must have heart disease, noncyanotic is preferable to cyanotic. This is like saying it is better to be able to breathe than not to be able to breathe.

One of the things I enjoy most about pediatric cardiology is its frequent use of multisyllable, multiword nomenclature spoken in a language last used two thousand years ago. Average medical phrases like "myocardial infarction," "pneumococcal pneumonia," "cerebrovascular accident," and "cardiopulmonary arrest" are confusing enough. The names used in peds cards, complete gibberish to laypeople and most non-baby heart docs alike, are much more impressive. "Patent ductus arteriosus" and "patent foramen ovale," for example, create "persistent fetal circulation," i.e., "the way the blood flowed while the baby was inside mommy is the way it is still flowing, and this is causing problems."

Picture a doctor addressing the parents of a newborn who failed to turn pink after birth. "Your baby probably has a PDA, uh, a patent ductus arteriosus, which has caused persistent fetal circulation. We've stabilized him for now but expect he'll have to go to the OR within twenty-four hours." Since many mommies and daddies have no idea what these entities are (including the "OR"), such a speech may create more than a little bit of anxiety.

Regardless, I'm delighted by such jargon. Imagine the majesty of gravely declaring, "I'm afraid this child has a ventricular septal defect," or, "Poor kid, he's got pulmonary and tricuspid atresia." Furthermore, I've discovered that any syndrome that isn't named in Latin is simply named after the doctor who first described it in the last century. This, of course, is even less descriptive of the actual condition.

"By God! I haven't seen a case of tetralogy of Fallot since '58!"

"Any fool can see that this is a straightforward case of Eisenmenger's syndrome. And you have the nerve to call yourself 'doctor'!"

"Unbelievable! This is the third kid with Ebstein disease I've seen this week!"

Dermatology, incidentally, is one of the few areas in medicine that effectively competes with pediatric cardiology for complexity and obscurity of nomenclature. Dermatologic conditions may include four or more terms having absolutely no meaning in plain English. A person with a bad chronic skin condition, for example, might be described as having "discoid psoriatic dermatitis with lichen planus chronicus and complexus." Really fantastic.

My patient was admitted at the age of nine months with complications resulting from surgery he'd had in the newborn period. He'd had cyanotic heart disease as a newborn, though I don't remember exactly what kind. In fact, being such a nice baby, it goes without saying that he had cyanotic heart disease. If he was a nasty, colicky, pissy little kid he couldn't possibly have been that sick.

During the prior operation, the surgeons had fiddled about with his aorta. He'd recovered from the surgery, gone home, and done well for a while, but after a few months he started to look and act sick again. His mommy said he'd get breathless very easily during feeding and, exhausted, fall asleep immediately afterward. He also tended to look a bit puffy at times. His general pediatric doctor noted that while he'd grown at a normal rate for a few months after surgery, his weight gain had recently slowed. Pediatric jargon describes such abnormally slow growth as "failure to thrive." There are many different possible causes for failure to thrive, but in this baby's case amazingly good odds backed its having something to do with his heart.

Mommy took her baby back to the ped heart docs. They immediately assumed grave expressions and got out their echocardiography machine to look at pictures of his heart. The echocardiography machine is a wonderful piece of technology that bounces sound waves around the inside of babies' chests, converts them to electric impulses, whisks them back and forth inside a computer, and displays them on a video screen as cross-sectional images of hearts. Plainly put, echocardiography translates as cross-sectional pictures of hearts "created by bouncing sound waves (echos)."

The pictures can be quite good. An actual heart cut in half and viewed cross-sectionally (a filthy exercise sometimes practiced by medical students) looks amazingly like the picture of the same cross-section seen on an echocardiography machine. It's a masterful piece of modern medical technology. It provides a tremendous amount of information without hurting in the least.

The peds cards people did an echocardiogram on Shorty (I nicknamed him Shorty because at nine months he was only the size of a three-month-old, though I didn't call him this in front of his mother) and discovered a small lump of scar tissue at the base of his aorta, right where he'd had the prior surgery. The peds cards docs called it a "shelf" of scar tissue. This shelf was bad for Shorty because, by narrowing his aorta, it forced his heart to strain when it pumped blood.

As an example, imagine blowing air through a short length of garden hose versus a straw. Because of its smaller diameter, much more effort is required to blow a given volume of air through the straw than the garden hose. Anyone forced to breathe through a straw would quickly get tired and red in the face from the effort.

Shorty's heart, working for a few months against the resistance caused by the shelf, had gotten tired, red in the face, and finally started to fail. Shorty was becoming a miniature Mr. Kram. His heart failure led to fluid buildup in his lungs and feet just as it had in the legendary ancient sundowner and chum of mine from thirty years back. This made him become short of breath easily (for example, while feeding) and gave him a puffy appearance. Heart failure also lowered his overall circulation. This was one reason he wasn't growing like a normal baby, that he was "failing to thrive." His itty-bitty little muscles and bones and intestines and brain, hungry and eager to grow, simply weren't getting enough blood to get strong and robust at the normal rate. Shorty had become a little baby with congestive heart failure.

The baby heart docs looked at Shorty's heart with the echocardiogram machine and told Shorty's mom, "Well, it looks like Shorty has developed a little shelf of scar tissue where they did the surgery and this is why he gets short of breath and looks puffy and isn't gaining weight as well as we'd want him to."

Shorty's mom, who was a beautiful, courageous young woman said, "What will happen, what will we have to do?"

The heart docs, being men and women of caution and restraint in these matters, said, "Well, right now we can control this problem with medications, but we'll have to keep a close eye on him [they would use sound waves to keep an eye on him]. It's possible that the shelf will get no bigger, but if it continues to grow and gets too big he might need another operation."

Shorty's mom burst into tears. After nine months her baby had developed a character, a personality that she loved very much. But, she also knew that she was being told the truth and agreed to these plans.

Shorty was started on the classic old-person medicine, Lasix. By making him pee, Lasix would prevent his getting overloaded with fluid that otherwise backed up behind his huffing, puffing heart, oozed and seeped into his lungs and feet, and made him short of breath and puffy. While the average older person might take 60, 80, 100, or more milligrams of Lasix every day, Shorty was placed on 5 mg, suspended in cherry-flavored syrup to make it more palatable for him. He went home and did well for a while.

Unfortunately, when he visited the baby heart docs every two weeks for echocardiography, they had to tell his mom that the shelf of scar tissue was getting bigger and bigger and his heart failure worse and worse. Finally, Shorty remained puffy and short of breath despite the use of Lasix at home, and had to be admitted to the hospital for larger, old-person-type Lasix doses, and supplemental oxygen.

His echocardiogram on admission showed the shelf, plain as day, extending three quarters of the way across his aorta, while his one-foot-square chest X ray showed how big, dilated, and puffed-out his resigned and tired nine-month-old heart had become in its battle with the scar tissue.

We put Shorty under an oxygen hood, a device made of clear plastic that looks like a miniature New York City water tower. The oxygen hood is open on the bottom and has a half circle cut out on one side. It fits snugly over the baby's head with room for his neck. A hose is attached to a nozzle on the hood, and fills it with oxygen for the baby to breathe. I put Shorty under a hood and turned on the oxygen. Having done this I was obligated to do a blood gas to ensure I had chosen an oxygen flow rate sufficient to meet his increased need. If you remember, a blood gas is a measurement of the oxygen content of arterial blood. It is taken to assess the adequacy of a patient's own breathing, or that of a respirator.

Shorty'd had around twenty or thirty blood gases after his original surgery. The spot on his wrist where I would stick the needle was totally covered with scars. Somewhere inside was his little, tiny radial artery, which, though small in a normal baby, was undoubtedly made even smaller by all the previous assaults. I took an itty-bitty little 26-gauge needle, not a whole lot bigger than a coarse hair, and stuck it into his itty-bitty little wrist right over the spot where I felt his itty-bitty little pulse, and poked it about in search of his itty-bitty little radial artery. After five or six sticks I still hadn't hit it and gave up. With each stick he'd get very upset and worried-looking, screw up his brow, sweat, and grunt, though he wouldn't cry. Crying made him too short of breath.

I cleaned up his wrist, which was covered with holes and spots of blood, and looked down at him. Both of us were covered with sweat and I yelled at him, "Where the hell is your goddam little artery, you little shit?! You think I like hurting you?" He was a pretty calm baby and knew a moment without pain was to be appreciated. When I finally stopped sticking him he simply stopped grunting and started to suck on his fingers, one of his favorite activities. I was so tired and pissed off that I wanted to pull his fingers out of his mouth and demand an answer, but I left his room and called my supervising resident to come and try to do the gas instead.

My supervising resident stuck him another five or six times and when she couldn't do it called the third-year who finally managed to get the blood.

After around the twelfth stick I'd wanted to say, "Listen, why don't we just tune up the oxygen all the way, and the hell with it, huh?" Unfortunately, sticking someone twelve or fifteen or twenty times creates a kind of self-feeding cycle of entrapment in which determination to succeed seems to outweigh the cost, even if the cost does not logically justify the result. Our assault on Shorty was our little Vietnam, we were determined to get the gas no matter what, like the United States was determined to stomp the commies no matter what, no matter how high the cost. So, I simply shut up, we got the blood, and thank Christ the amount of oxygen I had chosen was adequate so we wouldn't have to tune it up and repeat the gas.

Because I was the intern, all the senior people I'd called for help graciously allowed me to clean up the mess we'd made. There were at least twelve or fifteen little "butterfly" needles lying in the crib, all the paper, plastic, and garbage the needles were wrapped in, and spots of blood all over the place. I used a little guillotine machine to cut each needle from its hub. We used to do that to keep people from poking themselves and to prevent junkies from finding usable needles in the hospital garbage. We don't use them anymore since it's been discovered that the more people fiddle with needles the more likely they are to get stuck. Nobody wants to get stuck these days because of AIDS. Now we just drop the needles into big, hard, plastic containers, and don't fiddle with them at all. Someone with big, thick gloves collects the containers and incinerates them, which, I assume, kills all the AIDS germs. Incineration also prevents them from being useful to junkies.

I returned to Shorty's crib, cleaned him up, arranged his sheets to cover up the spots of blood, and left to attend to other tasks. About five minutes later a nurse went into his room and blew her top because blood was still visible on his sheets. She stormed up to me, demanding to know what kind of asshole would let a mom see her baby like that. The peds nurses were kind of intense.

I was still pissed off about the blood gas and being left to clean up, so I just said, "You should have seen him before I cleaned him up," and walked off. She stormed back into Shorty's room mumbling about what a bunch of insensitive assholes doctors were. I spent the rest of the day feeling hurt and persecuted.

The next day we had a big conference with Shorty's beautiful mom about his need for surgery. The pediatric cardiologists were there with their echocardiographs, as was the very intense pediatric cardiothoracic surgeon, a social worker, a few nurses, mom, a big box of Kleenex tissues, and me. The ped heart docs and surgeon immediately engaged mom in the Great Medical Hedge.

As you might remember, the Great Medical Hedge always has the same basic theme, "If we don't provide medical attention to your relative he will definitely die, and if we do he might die anyway, but he could also survive." Only the specifics of the kind of medical attention and the name of the patient vary. In Shorty's case they said, in essence, "If Shorty doesn't have the surgery he will certainly die before age two, and if he does have the surgery he will only probably die, but he also might do well." They couldn't even give her rough odds.

The social worker explained all the services that Shorty would get after his surgery, like home nurse and doctor visits, the nurses, assuming agonized expressions of sympathy and support, provided a continual stream of dry Kleenex tissues, and I sat silently, staring at the floor and twiddling my thumbs. Pediatrics people like to have big conferences where there is more of a comprehensive approach to a medical problem. At this conference there really wasn't a whole lot to say. Shorty would either definitely die, probably die, or possibly do well.

The problem was, as mom saw it, that she wasn't sure the torture of surgery and the postoperative period for Shorty was worth the outcome of his probably dying anyway. She loved him a lot and didn't think he had earned so much pain in his nine-month life. There was very little to reply to this. The M.D.'s repeated the Great Medical Hedge in varying forms a few times and then shut up while mom sniffled and the nurses fed her tissues in silence. The heart docs told her to take a few days to think about it and finally everyone shuffled out of the room.

I stayed behind after they left because mom was so

beautiful and I liked her company, because I was depressed and didn't want to go back to work, and because mom knew I was the person who'd had the most hands-on contact with Shorty and might want to know what I thought.

She said to me, "He's really a terrific baby, don't you think so?"

I'd actually had a few nice nontormenting moments with Shorty and even saw him smile once or twice. I agreed that he was a nice baby, a beautiful baby, and said, "Yes."

She told me about how the decision had been easier when Shorty was a newborn and she didn't know him so well, but now that he'd grown older and developed a personality she loved, the whole thing was much more difficult.

She said, "I want you to give me an answer, but I know you can't any more than any of the other people here can." I nodded. Then she straightened up, took in a great big sniff through her nose as people do when they feel it's time to stop crying, and said, "Well, I'll go tell them to go ahead and do the surgery." I nodded without even looking up from the floor.

She said, "You've been really nice through everything here and I want to thank you."

I was shaken by this because I hadn't done very much of anything except torment her kid and sit in the room staring at the floor, but I said, "You're welcome," and walked out quietly.

The next day they carted Shorty off to surgery. I went up to the pediatric intensive care unit to see him afterward, at the end of my last day of internship. He'd survived and was lying in his crib attached to a half-dozen monitors. He had a big bandage running down his chest, and one of the nurses was injecting morphine into his IV. I could tell he was in pain by his furrowed, worried, sweat-covered brow.

I said, "Hey, Shorty, how're you doing?" As usual, he

285

refused to answer and began to suck ferociously on his fingers. I left the pediatric ICU and began my first day as a resident the next morning on an adult medicine ward. I never saw Shorty or his mom again.

16

Moms and Babes

The obstetrics unit was the only place I worked in the hospital where human misery was not central to my job. I spent about six weeks there, watching wide-eyed as an endless succession of flushed, full to bursting mommies grunted and sweated and shrieked their progeny into the world. I'd never witnessed this process before, and was struck by its color, vigor, and high emotion. The glorious, shattering agony of childbirth, with its promise of life and health, was a welcome contrast to the stale, decaying misery I'd become so inured to on the Cloud Pavilion. I was dazzled by the vivid images and noise that flourished in the delivery room, the flood of bright red blood at the moment of birth, the flush of the laboring woman's face, the stunning volume of her bellows, and the sudden, brief quiet before the infant's first cry. The whole process had a rosiness to it, from the vitality of the mommies to the silence of their freshly swaddled babies, each exhausted from its recent tribulation, and still covered with the silky white dew of life in the womb.

The laboring women's amazing capacity for howling was a tribute to the health and hardiness that is the essence of normal childbirth. They made a stunning racket, behaving as though they were being physically torn apart (a description that is pretty close to the actual process of delivering a baby). To the experienced nurse or midwife this expressive agony was an important source of information on the progress of labor. Rapid-fire crescendo-decrescendo grunting and crying, for example, characterized a moderate early contraction, no cause for excitement, while a puretone, high-pitched, upper-decibel, all-out shriek might herald junior's imminent arrival, and warranted a quick check on mom's progress. There was a natural variation along this spectrum; some women maintained a pant and blow approach nearly to the end, while others commenced to yelping with the very first contraction. "Grand multiparas," our majestic title for women with as many as eight or more prior deliveries, addressed the task with resignation, while first-time mothers ("primiparas") became increasingly panicked with each contraction, and quickly lapsed into garbled recitations of the Lord's Prayer.

The nurses and midwives who worked on the labor and delivery floor (known in obstetrical circles as "L and D") were old hands at the baby biz and, other than its clinical import, regarded the anguish of delivering mommies casually or with indifference. Most were impervious to the clatter, and perked up an ear only when the windows began to rattle. The particularly wretched scream was even a source of gentle humor: "Lord have mercy! You'd think that woman was having a baby!" In the presence of mom and dad, of course, such frivolity was nowhere in evidence. The staff were good-hearted people who treated the patients and their families to theatrical expressions of grave sympathy, frequent whoops of encouragement, and copious helpings of tender loving care.

The openly lax attitude toward the tribulations of healthy, laboring women was a welcome respite from the dour hallways of the general medical floors. Similar flippancy was forbidden in that setting, where the business at hand was cancer, heart disease, and death. The agony of a mommy in labor, on the other hand, was a different story, and did not call for the tortured sympathy granted the medical patient. Labor pain resolved into relief, joy, and life, rather than continued pain and death, making our lack of compassion immediately forgivable, even to the most ethical and upright among us.

My rotation in labor and delivery was spent at NYG, which had a large midwifery service. This was unusual in New York, where high-powered, specialized medical care was the rule, and the skills of the generalist frowned upon. Obstetrics had a virtual monopoly on the business of childbirth, and midwifery, a formally licensed branch of nursing, was little recognized in the medical community. NYG was one of a small but growing number of institutions that acknowledged the skills of midwives, who also enjoyed a burgeoning popularity among the general public.

When I started my rotation I expected to find the two professions cooperating to provide complete care for the pregnant woman. After all, the labor floor was an oasis, a place in the hospital where the emphasis was on health rather than illness. Here, the business at hand was fundamentally optimistic, and would be devoid of the ill will that prevailed on the medical floors.

It took twelve seconds of working in the labor suite to set me straight. Incredibly, I'd totally forgotten the central focus of any form of hospital-based health care: politics, personality, and problems. The interaction between obstetricians and midwives, I discovered, was more a turf battle than a cooperative effort, and rarely without rancor.

The two professions approached childbirth completely differently. Midwives were left-wing and feminist, obstetricians Republican and conservative, and neither hesitated to criticize its counterpart. Midwives attacked OBs for their invasive methods and blunt bedside manners. OBs faulted midwives for not being sufficiently aggressive and placing style over outcome. Underneath, one wondered about less altruistic issues, like competition for business in an essentially static market. Not surprisingly, the conflict between the two provided an ongoing source of nastiness and amusement on the labor floor.

At NYG, the midwives did almost all of the deliveries. The obstetricians provided backup for those that became complicated, or holed up in the operating room doing gynecologic surgery and cesarean sections. At night, they withdrew to the on-call room, praying not to be paged. I spent most of my time learning about childbirth with the midwives, a very high-powered crowd of socially conscious women. As a doctor and a man, I was marked from the start. I rapidly discovered that the birth of a child was not a physical process, but a political event with wide-ranging social implications. The midwives enjoyed an apparently contractual right to politicize childbirth, and made regular, frenzied orations about medicine's perversion of this once natural process. The entire specialty of OB/GYN was a part of the ever evil White Man's use of technology to overpower and subjugate the masses. It was the oppression of women, plain and simple. Frequently, I bore sole responsibility for these lamentable facts, a burden I accepted in resigned silence.

Anyone who challenged the midwives' assertions found himself menaced by an avalanche of statistical reports clipped from a variety of nursing and midwifery journals. These articles, which had titles like "Nurse-Midwifery: The End of Obstetrics?" or "Cesarean Section: Medical Genocide?" documented irrefutably the hideous distortion of womanhood perpetrated by modern medicine.

A terse "Don't be stupid!" greeted those dumb enough to inquire about the benefits of surgery in childbirth. Of course, invasive methods are at times an unavoidable necessity. And, yes, many thriving bambinos would not have survived without the miracle of surgical delivery. That, the midwife declared, is not the point. The point is the over-application of technology in the process of "birthing," the loss of a woman's control over her own body, the loss of her ability to make decisions about her own care and fate, and the use of technology to benefit the doctor, rather than the patient. Or something like that.

"Birthing," the midwives' version of "labor," was sure to be heard dozens of times daily on the labor floor. It always reminded me of the scene in *Gone With the Wind* when the slave girl, faced with the delivery of a laboring heroine, shrieks, "A BABY! I don't know NOTHIN' about birthin' babies!"

Another big favorite with the midwives was the word "empower." To "empower," which had something to do with people controlling their own fate, was the pinnacle of the liberal midwife's aspirations. The term was held in almost mystical reverence and had very intense political and social overtones.

Though I wouldn't say it out loud, it seemed to me that midwives had more of a need for control than most would admit. True, the obstetrician's scalpel was much more emphatic than the midwife's "coaching." Still, I rarely saw a midwife let mom just do her thing, no Lamaze, no huffing and puffing: a raw delivery. The berserk, uncontrollable, full-speed-ahead, damn-the-torpedoes method of delivery frustrated the midwives, rendered furniture into kindling, ruptured eardrums, and distinctly redefined "empowerment." For the most part, however, this behavior (which was delicately termed "difficult") produced normal, bouncing babies, just like the ladies who sat stoically in bed, huffing and puffing, grunting and pushing exactly as they were told.

Junkies—surprise, surprise—were the most difficult women to deliver, and stretched the patience of even the most liberal midwives. Heroin and cocaine did not lend themselves to the empowerment of their victims. Being as bad with delayed gratification during childbirth as at any other time, laboring drug abusers flailed wildly about, kicking, screaming, punching, and ignoring all pleas for any degree of decorum, just as they did while withdrawing from drugs in the emergency room.

A junkie in lithotomy position (in the stirrups) was dangerously well poised to kick the deliverer—midwife or OB—squarely in the jaw. This once happened to me. I said, "Okay, now STOP PUSHING, and BREATHE!" Mommy shrieked, "YOU FUCKIN' BREATHE!" and the next thing I knew I was on the floor seeing stars. A midwife took over, kept her mouth shut, and mommy delivered her kid exactly as she pleased.

Unfortunately, the behavior of the drug abuser in labor was considerably more problematic than that of the uncooperative but healthy mom, because she often delivered a drug-addicted baby. These babies could develop trouble very quickly while still in the womb, and required constant monitoring during labor. This was a difficult task when mom was savagely swinging at everyone in sight.

The obstetricians had no apologies about controlling labor and delivery, and the likely outcome of their approach, empowering or not. Methods used to monitor the progress of labor and baby's well-being, for example, ranged from those of the absolutely most liberal midwives to those of OBs who'd keep a scalpel in the glove compartment of their cars, just in case. In the least invasive approach, the midwife simply listened to mom's belly for baby's pulse during contractions, differing patterns suggesting differing degrees of fetal health. I never saw this done without a stethoscope, but imagine that in the ultimate of empowerment, the midwife merely plastered her ear against mom's belly, listening for the faint, rapid, pitter-patter. The usual method was to strap a microphone around mom's middle that provided a continual readout of the infant's heart rate. The scalpel-in-the-glove-compartment OBs, on the other hand, could read signs of "fetal distress" into a moderate case of maternal hiccups, and screw a wire right through the cervix into baby's head (a "scalp electrode"), plugging his pulse directly into a video display. Sometimes this resulted in the plugging of mommy into the video by mistake, giving everyone a big scare when it appeared that baby's heart rate was about half normal.

The ultimate in obstetrical aggression was the cesarean section (or "C-section"). There is little that is more controlling than putting mommy to sleep, cutting her belly open, and manually removing her baby. Not much in the way of empowerment, either. I didn't get involved with surgical obstetrics at all except to go to the operating room to watch whenever there was a C-section. Most were "crash" sections, emergency surgery accomplished in a blur of metal and blood. Normal labor could sour quickly, in seconds or minutes, prompting the OBs to scatter "process" to the breeze and reach pronto for a knife. It seemed to me that most sections were done when baby couldn't handle labor anymore and simply began to poop out ("fetal distress"). Speed was essential to get the ailing babe into the soothing arms of pediatricians who, looking very uncomfortable in surgical masks, waited quietly nearby, armed with fantastically small intubation equipment for use if baby was too tired to breathe on his own. The whole scene was very dramatic.

Cesarean sections were also performed on an elective basis. One condition necessitating planned "abdominal delivery," for example, was placenta previa, in which an abnormally positioned placenta covered the opening to the

293

cervix within the uterus. Because the cervix had to open for junior to make his exit during labor, this situation created a considerable dilemma for those favoring natural childbirth. Mom might bleed to death and junior lose his supply of oxygenated blood. Pregnant women with placenta previa had to live in the hospital for the last few months of their pregnancies because of the risk of sudden vaginal bleeding, and undergo surgical delivery at term. There were all sorts of criteria to certify that baby was ripe for delivery, and everyone waited with bated breath to see if he'd be able to breathe on his own once he was outside the womb.

I did fewer than fifty deliveries as an intern, a drop in the bucket in terms of becoming even vaguely competent. My own approach to childbirth differed from that of both the OBs and the midwives, and combined awe, bewilderment, and terror. Messing up on the average medical patient could be bad, but ruining a delivery seemed totally different. To me it was the worst possible medical mistake that could be made, akin to accidentally running over a woman with a baby carriage or burning down an orphanage. The idea that some poor kid might spend the rest of his life with cerebral palsy or mental retardation because I screwed up was absolutely terrifying. It helped me understand why the OBs were so focused on outcome over style. It was their necks that were on the line no matter who screwed up. Lawsuits over blown deliveries could be incredibly vicious, and if it was a midwife who'd messed up it was only because an OB had allowed her to do so.

I wouldn't even consider doing a delivery without a midwife or OB looking over my shoulder at all times. Even then I didn't relax, though I loved doing them. The intensity and emotion and color consumed me completely, and

I'd find myself drenched with sweat and shaking after each one. For the first few deliveries I had absolutely no idea at all what was going on, and did exactly what I was told. I was petrified at the idea of bending and twisting an emerging kid in the wrong directions, and having him come out tied in a knot. The midwives were the best teachers, whispering when to instruct mom to push, when to tell her to relax, and when to get tough and start barking instructions.

One of the midwives was terrifically easygoing and straightforward. She took me through several deliveries, watching over my shoulder and offering instructions in her heavy Chinese accent as though I were working my way through a car engine.

In one delivery an infant had reached the point where, normally, his head would turn just before emerging. The midwife instructed me to help the process along, saying, "Okay. Now you help turn his head."

Being as gentle as possible I clumsily attempted to turn the child's head, but met resistance. She again leaned to my ear and, unhurried, whispered, "I think you turn wrong way. Maybe you try other direction."

I did so, and the child's head popped right out. She leaned back, smiling, and patted me on the back. "See?! Easy!"

I did several memorable deliveries, including that of a woman who'd had five or six previous kids, didn't like hospitals, and decided to wait until the last possible moment to `come in and deliver her most recent. She came waddling onto the labor floor like someone in desperate need of a toilet, red in the face, and grasping her crotch in an apparent attempt to prevent her baby from spilling out onto the floor. We threw her onto a bed where she gave a great big heave and delivered her child all at once. The fantastic part about it was that I didn't even have time to put on a pair of sterile rubber gloves. I ran my hands under a faucet and leapt across the room to catch the baby bare-handed. What a feeling! All that hot, slippery blood and ooze all over my hands and forearms and spattered on my shirt and face, and the wriggling, living, breathing infant squirming against my naked skin. It was wonderful.

In another memorable delivery, mom had progressed all the way to crowning without breaking the amniotic sac. Put differently, her baby's head was bulging from her vagina (crowning) and the "bag of water" (the fluid-filled amniotic sac in which the infant develops) still had not broken. The tissue-thin membrane of the sac protruded about six inches in front of the kid, tense and straining with fluid. My face was no more than three feet away when it finally burst, and I was drenched with the steamy, hot, clear fluid. I was tempted to try a little taste, but managed to restrain myself.

One of my favorite parts in a delivery was the reaction of the father, especially the first-time daddy. Perhaps being a man I was best able to empathize with men, but it was daddy's reaction that touched me the most, like when big six-foot bruisers watched dumbfounded and then burst into tears on baby's arrival. I never saw a daddy behave badly, the worst behavior being an inability to do anything more than gaze awestruck as mommy struggled. Most were incredibly attentive to their wives (or "partners," the 1980s version of "lover" that does not specify marital status — or sex), at times withstanding significant verbal abuse.

"You BASTARD!! You did this to me!! I'm going to KILL you when this is over!"

"Take your hands off of me! Get out, OUT, OUT, OUT! Goddam you! I never want to see you again, you SON OF A BITCH!"

It was also wonderful fun to turn to the first-time father

after the delivery and congratulate him, calling him "Dad," and watch his eyes bug out at the implications of that title. Another favorite was, "We only take out what you put in," a reference to the fact that it is the sperm cell that determines the sex of the child.

Sometimes I even allowed dad to cut the umbilical cord, a deed fraught with Freudian implications. Many refused, and those who accepted had to be reassured every step of the way.

"Cut it there!"

"Yes, right there!"

"Go ahead, cut!"

"Yeah!! Perfect!!"

One of the most interesting aspects of working at NYG was the significant population of Southeast Asian refugees living in the area immediately adjacent to the hospital. These people added a unique cultural diversity to the hospital's patient load, and demonstrated completely different attitudes and emotional responses to health and disease. I had many Southeast Asian clinic patients, including a number of Cambodian women for whom I provided prenatal care. Plucked from squalid refugee camps and deposited ignominiously in the tenements of the promised land, these women negotiated childbirth completely differently from their Western counterparts. In contrast to virtually all pregnant American women, they exhibited a remarkable stoicism during labor. The midwives' scream-classification system had no bearing with Cambodians, who remained almost completely silent throughout. A barely audible grunt usually meant the kid was already halfway out. Many of the staff were inexperienced with these ways and awaited the normal signs of active labor. This risked the embarrassment of peeking in to check on mom's progress, only to find her quietly breast-feeding her still-wet newborn.

One night, one of my Cambodian patients went into labor while I was working on the delivery floor. She arrived alone, silent, and in active labor. Although the hospital employed a few bilingual Cambodians, no one was present at night to translate. I could say about four sentences in Khmer as a result of an abortive attempt two years earlier to learn the language, and she spoke no English at all. I tried saying, "Which way to the nearest restaurant?" but got the tonality all wrong. I'm sure she'd have been happy to follow my instructions/coaching; the difficulty arose from the fact that, lacking guidance or understanding of the Western medical role in childbirth, she simply did things her own way. Hers was the most natural delivery I ever saw. At one point, five nerve-wracking minutes after she managed to mime her need for a toilet, a midwife and I discovered the tiny woman doing her absolute best to deliver her kid right into the bowl. We put her back in bed and simply stood back while she delivered her baby. All I could do was catch. I don't care what the midwives say, the purest form of a woman controlling her own body is when she delivers her baby her own way. No instructions, and no knives.

It almost killed me when my new Cambodian mommy patient asked me to name her brand-new little boy, her first American citizen. Here was this woman all alone in this big, ugly city after all the horrors of the war in Southeast Asia and years in refugee camps, whose husband, through some horrendous, mindless bureaucratic blip, was still rotting on the Thai-Cambodian border dodging Vietnamese artillery, and she was trusting me to make the right decision for her baby in his spanking new life in this frightening and noisy country. I discovered through a translator that she wanted a Western name for her boy, the better to help him get along in America. I thought about it almost exclusively for days and days, especially fearful that

I'd accidentally render him vulnerable to the kind of name taunting so enjoyed by school-aged boys, and finally came up with "David." "David" lent his full name a soft musical cadence. The entire episode was probably my greatest accomplishment as an intern.

Because I delivered, or rather caught, David when I was an intern, I had the privilege of giving him his vaccinations and plotting his growth on the pediatric growth chart and treating his sniffles and ear infections over the next two years of my residency. He was a welcome respite from the hospital and when he graduates from college I'm going to tell him, "Kid, I knew you when. Yes, I did."

17

Other Matters of
the Crotch

America is shocked, dismayed, and concerned by the phenomenon of teenage pregnancy. I'm dismayed and concerned, but not so shocked. I don't find it so shocking in a society that so defies the well-muscled buttock that many kids say, "Well, what the heck?!" and hop in the sack. Teenagers are not known for their restraint. Combine this fact with stupefying irresponsibility, limitless overeager sperm, lush, blossoming fertility, and immeasurable libido, and a new human is certain to be conceived. Shocking? Not really.

One of the most important parts of my job in the clinic was the prevention of teenage pregnancy. A never-ending battle against the union of juvenile sperm and egg cells. Teens who came in complaining of sore throats and fevers left with diaphragms and oral contraceptive pills, lectured mightily on the sorrows of unplanned pregnancy. One unwanted birth successfully prevented was a victory as satisfying as any medical cure.

I started my job as invisible bedroom chaperon in traditional liberal form, engaging my adolescent charges in the most adultlike negotiations, open expressions of feeling and concern culminating in handshakes and mutually agreeable solutions. These discussions, through unknown mechanisms, acted as potent fertility agents, virtually guaranteeing follow-up visits for prenatal care. Young women paraded from my office unshakably committed to the iron-fisted control of their own fertility, only to march back in the healthful flush of pregnancy, fraught with questions about morning sickness, vitamins, and Lamaze classes. Suspecting a problem, I reevaluated my style of contraception guidance. Outright manipulation, combining a light touch with insidious directness, might work much better.

The counseling method that proved most effective was when I'd face the patient directly, away from my desk, draping myself casually with elbows on knees to rid the atmosphere of any apparent rank. In this carefully arranged scene I am the model of impartiality, a doctor in name only.

"So, now that we've dealt with your sore throat, lemme ask you, have you done any thinking about contraception?" My tone is casual and easygoing.

The patient, a girl of fifteen who is still teary-eyed from an extensive exam with a tongue depressor, hopes only to take leave of this oddball as quickly as possible. She is regarding me at an angle, eyebrows raised, and wipes her nose with her sleeve. "Huh?"

I slump backward and dangle my arms loosely over the back of the chair. My face is pure sincerity. "You know, birth control."

The patient glances at the door. She understands exactly what I'm referring to, but doesn't want to talk about it.

"What?"

"Birth control."

"What's that?"

"That's you and your boyfriend making sure you don't get pregnant when you have sex." I am still relaxed, but my approach is direct, no-nonsense.

The patient is suddenly abashed. She stares at the floor. "Uh . . . we don't do none a that."

"None of what, sex or birth control?"

301

"What you said."

"Birth control?"

"Yeah."

"Well, have you thought about it?"

The patient doesn't want to get in trouble with the doctor. "My boyfriend, he said don't worry about that."

"Why not?"

"He said don't worry about it."

"Does he use a condom?"

"What?"

"A rubber. Does he use a rubber?"

"Oh, he said he can't use none a that."

"Why not?"

"He said he don't need it."

My demeanor is changing from casual to serious. I am again leaning on my knees, my head protruding toward the patient to impress upon her the import of the issue. My forehead is wrinkled with concern. The patient is now playing with her fingernails, which are covered with chipped red nail polish.

"Let me ask you this. Do you want to get pregnant?"

The patient looks away from her hands and resumes an intense scrutiny of the floor. Her right knee is bouncing up and down at high speed. The possibility of pregnancy is ever present but dim in her mind. She halfheartedly assumes it will not happen to her, and does nothing to prevent it. She cannot challenge her boyfriend's hollow reassurance that birth control isn't necessary, and knows he will not use condoms. It's easiest for her to avoid considering the issue altogether, and she doesn't like having it forced into the open. She will now become contrary and vague, refusing to admit to her concerns.

"I don't know."

"Well, if you and your boyfriend are having sex without doing anything to keep from having a baby, that means you must want a baby, right?" I'm giving her a chance to remain ornery while admitting she doesn't want to get pregnant.

She takes a tentative nibble and then backs off. "No . . . but, if that happens . . . besides, my boyfriend said don't worry about it."

I am no longer negotiating, but forcing reality on the patient. I allow a shade of exasperation into my voice.

"Let me ask you this. Do you have any girlfriends who have babies?"

"Yeah."

"And were they doing anything to keep from getting pregnant?"

"I don' know." Sullen. The patient sees where I am leading the discussion and feels trapped. "How'm I supposed to know? I wasn't in bed with them." She knows very well, but will not admit that she is making the same mistake that led to her friends' pregnancies. I ignore her response, clarifying this fact.

"And are their boyfriends doing anything to help them take care of their babies?"

"I don' know that neither . . . yeah, some are." Slightly less sullen, predisposed to agree with a criticism about boys.

"And do your girlfriends tell you how hard it is to take care of a baby?"

"No." (Yes.)

"And do some of them drop out of school?"

"No." (Yes.)

"And do you want to go to college after you graduate from high school?"

"I don' know." (Yes.)

"And are you going to get an abortion when you get pregnant?" *When* you get pregnant.

"I don' know." (Probably not.)

"And when you have a baby, are you going to bring it to class with you in college, or to your job, or maybe your boyfriend will take care of it?" *When* you have a baby.

"I don' know."

I straighten up and turn my chair to face my desk. The point is made and if I push it any more the patient will refuse my next offer. I smile to indicate that I'm not angry and my tone shifts to the matter-of-fact.

"So, listen. I think you're a smart young woman and you know that not using birth control really isn't such a good idea. I understand that you like your boyfriend, but maybe he's not as smart as you, and you have some things to do before you start fooling with babies. Right?" I have complimented the patient, allied myself with her against her boyfriend who, as she knows deep inside, is lying, and allowed her to accept the idea of birth control as her own decision.

"I guess so."

"So, what I'm going to do is tell you about the kinds of birth control you can use. Your boyfriend won't even know you're using it. That way you can make sure yourself that you don't get pregnant. Then you can go to college or get a job or do whatever you want when you're finished with high school without worrying about taking care of a baby." Empowerment.

I bullied dozens of adolescent girls into accepting the idea of contraception in exactly this manner. In my initial liberal approach I'd made the mistake of sending them off with a handful of pamphlets describing different methods of birth control, not seeing them again until the third month of pregnancy. Now, having felt the tug, I made sure to set the hook.

There was no question that oral contraception was the only method with half a chance of success for the average teenage girl. The IUD was out for this age group, and the diaphragm far too complicated. The few who opted to try it gave up almost immediately. I learned to say, "I'll tell you about the diaphragm if you like, but I really think the pill is going to be the best method for you. Do you know anything about it?"

Most girls had several concerns, ranging from its imagined capacity to cause unwanted hair growth to the possibility of instantaneous death with the first dose. I addressed each of these carefully, emphasized that the risks were far smaller than those of unwanted pregnancy or abortion, and explained all the signs of possible trouble. I even drew elaborate diagrams of the dose schedule.

"You start on the *first* Sunday after your next period begins. That means that if your period starts on Monday, Tuesday, Wednesday, Thursday, Friday, or Saturday, you start taking the pills on Sunday, and if it starts on Sunday you take the first pill on the *same day*. Then you take one pill *every day*. Understand?"

When I was certain the patient could repeat these instructions, I gave her a congratulatory handshake and sent her off with two free packets and a prescription for several months more. Most incredibly, some patients even decided to use them.

Many others, however, didn't pay any attention at all, and wound up on L and D nine months later.

I delivered several adolescent girls. Being children, most behaved badly, ignored my instructions, cried uncontrollably, and were a nuisance in general. One, a girl of fourteen, progressed to the point that her baby was all but delivered and then started to scream, cry, and refuse to do any more pushing. The midwife who was assisting in the delivery had strapped a monitor on mom's belly, providing a readout of the baby's pulse. So-called decelerations, periodic decreases in the fetal pulse rate, were the usual means of evaluating the infant's health, a sustained and progressive drop suggesting fetal distress. Naturally, it was right at the moment that mom refused to cooperate that junior's pulse began a steady decline.

I tried the friendly approach. "Okay! You're doing

great! Just one more good push and you're finished! You can do it!" Pulse rate 110.

"I CAN'T, I CAN'T, I CAN'T, I CAN'T, LEAVE ME ALONE, NOOOO!" No pushing.

I tried the authoritarian approach, advocated by experts in adolescent medicine. "Now listen to me carefully. It is time for you to deliver your baby, and I won't have any more of this. You are perfectly capable of pushing one more time and you must do so right now." Pulse rate 90.

"NO, NO, NO, NO, NO, NOOOOOO! I CAN'T. AHHHHH!" No pushing. Pulse rate 60.

I would have to resort to terror. I picked up a sterile scissors and brandished it in front of mommy's face. "I'M GOING TO CUT YOU RIGHT NOW." Scissors move purposefully toward crotch.

"NOOOOOOOOOOOOO!!!!!" Tremendous push, and a bouncing baby boy pops into my hands. Baby and mom do fine.

The diaphragm, incidentally, was great fun to teach to women who were older and more reliable. I had a cross-sectional model of the female reproductive tract in my office, made especially to show how the diaphragm fit. I'd demonstrate on the model and then get the patient up in the stirrups (correct liberal phrase, "footrests") and guide her through the process of inserting and removing the device. I used a Vaselinelike lubricant to mimic contraceptive jelly, which I called "goop."

"Remember, you have to put the goop on to kill all the sperm. Ask for 'contraceptive jelly' at the drugstore. That's contraceptive jelly, and not grape jelly or strawberry jelly." Every once in a while you'd hear about someone smearing Welch's on her diaphragm and wondering why she got pregnant.

Once I'd shown the patient how to use the diaphragm

correctly I'd ask her to do it herself. Some women were too shy to do so while I was watching, so I'd turn my back and then check to make sure it was in right. Others took to the task with gusto, brows furrowed. The goop made the diaphragm so greasy and slippery that it was almost impossible to grasp. It frequently went flying across the room, providing lots of comic relief. The occasional victim, unable to remove the contraption, became panicky. I'd say, "Just reach in there, hook your finger underneath and pull it on out!" After much struggling the patient met success, displaying the diaphragm like a prize trout as we laughed together. Amazingly, some even went on to use it.

I did very, very little contraception counseling with adolescent boys, mostly because I rarely saw them as patients. Those I did see, full of ego, semen, and libido, refused to consider using a condom, virtually the only form of contraception (aside from vasectomy) available to men. Unfortunately, the long-term sequelae of irresponsible sex in juvenile males were far less forbidding than pregnancy, leaving me little ammunition for bullying these patients. Even outright lies about the possibility of getting AIDS through unprotected heterosexual intercourse elicited little response. With boys, I usually took care of the sore throat and sent the patient off into the world.

Matters of the crotch extend far beyond the perils of pregnancy and childbirth. Sex accounts for a cornucopia of other predicaments in both the male and female groin, from the trivial to the life threatening. Gynecology, the science of female troubles from the ovaries to the escutcheon, accounts for a large percentage of the average general practice, and an even bigger chunk of emergency room visits. As an intern and resident I did about a million pelvic exams for assorted problems where the sun don't shine, and most such woe was the direct consequence of physical congress between the sexes.

The list of sexually transmitted diseases (STDs), long and impressive, extends far beyond entities like AIDS and herpes, the favorites of the popular media. Chlamydia trachomatis, a little known yet highly precocious bacterium, shows a particular predilection for the reproductive tract and is currently running neck and neck with herpes simplex type II ("genital herpes") at the head of the STD pack. The cause of drippy dicks, infections of the cervix, uterus and fallopian tubes, chronic belly pain, infertility, and neonatal eye infections and pneumonia, chlamydia has a special inclination for the less than responsible "sexually active" adolescent, and can be grown from 20 to 25 percent of inner-city teenage groins. This happy circumstance has several causes. For one thing, the critter is quite tricky, and often fails to cause the classic symptoms of the clap, fiery pee-pee in males, and sloppy, itchy pubes in females. Further, it is not addressed by organized control efforts or reportable to the health department (as are gonorrhea and syphilis). Combine these factors with a sexual mode of transmission, and an infection will spread unchecked. Chlamydia has become a bona fide epidemic in less than ten years.

Gonorrhea, the classic cause of the drip, is once again on the move after more than a decade of decline that ended in the late 1970s/early 1980s. Herpes, the first of a lengthening list of permanent sexual stigmata, has recently been bumped as front-runner in general popularity and awareness by AIDS. "The big A," as we know all too well, is the first STD of the antibiotic era that is both incurable and deadly. Syphilis, a rarity in the 1970s, found almost solely among promiscuous homosexual men, has also jumped in prevalence in the last decade. Recently, it has shown signs of becoming epidemic among inner-city "crack" abusers.

Other sexually transmitted diseases, though less common, are equally fascinating. Chancroid, the cause of pitted, ragged, painful genital ulcers, is sure to be seen at least once or twice a month in the ER, and must be carefully distinguished from the painless "chancre" of primary syphilis. "Genital warts," the result of infection by human papilloma virus (HPV), have been related to abnormal Pap smears and can besmirch even the handsomest of external genitalia.

It should be no surprise that sexually transmitted diseases chiefly afflict the young. Just the same, I was amazed by the range of sexual goings-on, and subsequent morbidity, among children thirteen and fourteen years old. The victim of archaic social sensibilities, I was actually shocked by the extensive pregnancy histories and procreative vigor of girls who had yet to graduate from the ninth grade.

Pelvic inflammatory disease (PID), an infection of the uterus and fallopian tubes almost always caused by sexually transmitted organisms, was the most common single cause for admission of adolescent girls at MH. Less than responsible young girls, engaging in less than responsible acts with less than responsible young boys, found their cervices rudely colonized by a variety of critters, particularly gonorrhea and chlamydia. Once safely ensconced, the organisms enjoyed a brief period of respite and percolation before taking exploratory excursions into the uterus and tubes where they'd percolate some more before establishing a full-blown, painful infection.

It only took a half hour working in the ER to learn that the first thing you had to think of in a young female with pain in the lower belly was pelvic inflammatory disease. This always called for a pelvic exam, the centerpiece of the gynecologist's trade, and a major ordeal in a child of fourteen, involving a great deal of crying, squirming, and refusing to cooperate. In a kid there were only two ways to approach it. One was to say, "Okay, get on the table and let's get this over with and don't fight with me because the more you fight the longer it's going to take," and the other was to get extremely involved, explaining exactly what you were going to do, and how trying to relax was extremely important, and don't be embarrassed because every woman has to go through it, and if I hurt you just tell me and I'll stop what I'm doing, and the rest of it.

After twelve hours in the ER, six heart attacks, four seizures, eleven overdoses, two suicide attempts, and four prior fifteen-year-olds with lower belly pain, this could become a little tiring and you'd want to say, "If you're so friggin' shy about your pussy how the hell did you wind up with PID to start with?"

I have to say that the liberal method of doing a pelvic was the best in terms of keeping the patient relaxed and completing the exam quickly and comfortably. My approach combined the folksy and straightforward. I'd help the patient into the stirrups, tilt the headrest up so she could see my face, and say, "I'll place my hand on your thigh for a moment and then on the outside of your vagina. I'm telling you this so that you won't be startled when I examine you." According to the liberals, neutral words like "examine" and "place" were to be used instead of those like "touch" and "feel," which might have sexual connotations. The whole idea of sexual connotations while a patient was in the stirrups struck me as ridiculous, but there are a lot of weirdos in medicine.

The first part of the exam was an inspection of the external genitalia. The next part was putting in the speculum, which was necessary for examination of the cervix, Pap testing, and cultures. This always caused a big ruckus in the bashful teenager, many of whom snapped their vaginas shut with vise-like force, demonstrating frightening strength of the pelvic and perineal musculature. Sometimes I'd manage to distract the patient by promising her a peek at the cervix with a mirror, dimly portraying the organ as "a nose between your vagina and womb." Many an adolescent girl (and adult woman) jumped at this opportunity, changing the tone of the exam from embarrassment and discomfort to curiosity and learning. Feminist publications, ordaining back-of-the-hand familiarity of every woman with her own cervix as an absolute political and social obligation, even diagram the contorted means by which each lady may insert and position her own speculum and mirror for this purpose.

The second part of the pelvic was the "bimanual exam." By putting two fingers into the vagina and under the cervix with one hand and pressing down just above the pelvis with the fingers of the opposite hand, the examiner could feel the uterus and adjacent fallopian tubes and ovaries. The key physical finding for PID in the pelvic was "cervical motion tenderness." Using the two "intravaginal" fingers, I'd jiggle the cervix and carefully observe the patient for signs of intense pain. I assumed that agitating the cervix in this way caused the uterus to move, and that an infected uterus was sensitive to motion. Cervical motion tenderness (CMT) could be marked, resulting in the "chandelier sign" (i.e., the patient was so tender she flew off the table and wound up hanging from the chandelier).

At worst, a properly done pelvic was limited to physical pain without embarrassment, while a good one became a learning experience for the patient. At the very least, I considered it an achievement to get through the exam on a fourteen-year-old without a ton of tears, wailing, and bucking around on the table.

The management of PID varied depending on the facility. At MH, age was critical in the decision to admit a patient for PID because of its potential to muck up subsequent pregnancies. Improperly treated, it could lead to scarring of the fallopian tubes, infertility, and ectopic ("tubal") pregnancy. A woman so afflicted could nail the hospital to the wall in a lawsuit. Thus, a fourteen-year-old with a so-so, maybe/maybe not case of PID wound up on the adolescent ward getting a week of IV antibiotics and comparing notes with her roommates, while the thirty-year-old needed a hot, pus-laden, writhing, roaring case to get admitted. If you couldn't see the uterus glowing and pulsating beneath the skin the admission was considered "soft." Most of the postadolescent young women with PID were sent home with a shot in the butt, a prescription for oral antibiotics that they might or might not get filled, and the heartfelt command to "feel better and come back in three days if you're still having pain."

Generally speaking, the consequences of ill-advised sexual relations in males were much less involved than those in women. The notable and obvious exception was found among gay men, who only a few years ago faced the possibility of extinction from AIDS. Though education and behavioral changes have now obviated this prospect, the same fate currently faces several million drug abusers (which is a completely different subject).

I saw many, *many* guys for crotch problems, 95 percent of whom had straightforward drippy dick: chlamydia and gonorrhea. They received the same treatment as their (postadolescent) female counterparts, a shot in the ass, a prescription, and a pat on the back.

Most men were seen in the ER, treated, and released. In three years at MH, I saw one guy with an infection of the prostate who needed admission out of about three hundred guys with itchy dicks, and his problem wasn't even sexually transmitted.

One of the best parts about treating men was that, being male, it was permissible to make bad sexist jokes, and I rarely missed a chance to do so. While I'd never describe a female patient as having an "itchy twat," I made regular declarations regarding "itchy dicks," "drippy dicks," "sore dicks," "male problems," "GC in the pee-pee," (from gonococcus, the cause of gonorrhea), "fire in the hole," etc. Sometimes, when a coworker asked, "What's your patient got?" I'd simply clap my hands, smiling. I also had no trouble getting directly to the point in the male exam, and felt no need to be apologetic or folksy in my approach. Saying "Pull down your pants and underpants and lie on the table, face up" was liberal enough. Though not nearly as emphatic as a pelvic, the male exam did involve mucking about with the patient's penis and testicles and, under the guise of checking the prostate, included a rectal for extra cruelty. Overall, it could be very uncomfortable. Still, if a patient became nervous or shy I'd just say, "Hold still. I'll be done in about thirty seconds."

I was equally less apologetic about the probable origin of the problem. When patients asked, "What do you think, Doc?" the answer was, "I think you had sex with one woman too many," or something equally disrespectful. It was almost a guarantee that it was the guy who'd been messing around, rather than his partner. Sometimes guys swore to absolute monogamy for a good five minutes before confessing to "this one chick." Others chortled and shrugged, seeking my approval of their virility.

Though it was none of my business how they'd gotten the infection, I enjoyed the chance to pry into other men's sex lives under the guise of professionalism. The correct liberal approach, for the sake of completeness, went as follows: "The most likely cause of the pain or discharge you experience when you urinate is a sexually transmitted disease. I'll have no problem treating it, but you must bring in your partner or partners to be treated for this as well." I preferred to say, "You've got the drip, and I don't think your wife or girlfriend is going to be too pleased about it," which felt much more honest.

One guy, knowing exactly what he had, actually brought along his pregnant wife, knowing she also would need treatment. I raked him over the coals, no holds barred.

"The very least little tiny bit of respect you could've shown your wife if you were going to fuck around would've been not to fuck her afterwards, full well understanding that giving her the clap could be a very big problem in pregnancy. That was a real asshole maneuver, big guy." He gave me a big smile and chortle and announced that he just couldn't help himself, right there in front of his ripe little wife. I agree with the feminists, guys like that should have their dicks cut off.

Now that we have AIDS, I lecture (heterosexual) men that they are putting themselves at risk for the disease by being promiscuous. Because the risk of a man getting AIDS from unprotected heterosexual intercourse is relatively low (that's *relatively* low, and not "insignificant"—I do not want to be accused of encouraging unsafe sex practices), this is just a ploy to try to keep them from spreading easily transmittable diseases, like gonorrhea, chlamydia, and herpes.

One guy brought his girlfriend into the ER for a runny groin. After examining her I sat them both down for a quick lecture. I said, "You know, with AIDS running around it's a bit risky to have sex outside of your relationship with each other. It's really much safer to be monogamous."

They both listened very intently, and then the guy shook his head in vigorous agreement. "Oh, don't worry, Doc, we always have sex inside." I pursed my lips, nodded, walked out of the room, and asked the nurse to give 'em both a shot in the butt and send 'em on their merry way.

Several of the nurses I worked with loved to treat men for drippy dicks because it meant they could punish them with a needle. The use of penicillin to treat gonorrhea involved two tremendous shots, one in each buttock of a thick, oily preparation that hurt like hell. Gonorrhea, however, plays cat and mouse with the medical profession, developing resistance to the drugs used for treatment.

314

Penicillin is now considered inadequate for 100-percent cure, and the bug has started to show traces of resistance to the newer drugs. Unfortunately for the nurses, ceftriaxone, the latest, is much less painful than the old shot of penicillin.

Male patients, even big, ugly guys, could get very skittish about injections. They'd say, "So, Doc, what're you gonna do? Like, do I have to get a shot for this?" I'd say, "Yep," and they'd go, "Oh, man!" and start squirming like little kids. Then they'd say, "Where?" and I'd reply, "Where do you think," intimating that it would naturally have to be in the penis, the site of the problem. They'd jump off the stretcher, saying, "Oh, SHIT! No way!" I'd smile. "Only kidding. You'll get the shot in the ass, and you better hope the nurse is nice about it."

Despite all of the frustrations, I enjoyed treating people for sexually transmitted diseases. It provided the chance to make a clean, tight diagnosis, to treat with the possibility of cure, and even to get into some good, old-fashioned patient counseling. Most incredibly, most patients didn't die! True, most did go out and get infected all over again, and true, medicine is being overwhelmed by the epidemic interaction between sex and drugs: orgies in crack houses, junkies with AIDS, and the like. Still, when I saw a guy with the drip, I could cure him. As a preceptor of mine used to say, "Do one good thing for one person each day, and that is enough." And I left it at that.

Epilogue

Friends of mine who are doctors read my book and got pissed off. They said, "Christ! You make it sound as if we never do a bit of good for anyone! Do you think that's an honest message to project to the reading public?" Fascinated by the idea of a "reading public," I sat down to give this criticism a good think. Incredibly, it is true that a few of my patients actually felt better as a result of my ministrations, even the intentional ones. Like the occasional kiddie with an earache who felt better with a few doses of ampicillin and two spoons of kiddie's Tylenol. There are even one or two guys who are alive because I happened to be at the right place at their worst time, snatching them from the brink with my ever sure, gentle hands. I assume that at this very moment they are laughing and loving, eating and drinking, walking and talking, and burglarizing people's houses, just as they did before we met. It's a great feeling.

So, I thought about the whole thing for about four minutes and decided, "What the hell, the reading public can think whatever they want." Besides, I'm really in no mood to get into a major rewrite. No one gave Joseph Heller a hard time for failing to portray the more positive aspects of World War II, so why should I have to be so fair about medicine?

Nonetheless, medicine has become a very different endeavor for me since the days of internship, and my feelings about it have changed significantly. The truth is that all of the anecdotes I've described about internship and the treatment of patients are true, both the heartwarming and the horrible; only the names and places have been changed to protect the guilty. Money and politics remain the chief motivating forces in medicine, and doctors who wish primarily to serve their patients are forced to work in this framework.

Fact is, though, that all the nonsense aside, medicine remains an intensely powerful means of doing good in people's lives. It's clear to me that I lack the energy even to try to change the system, and it's unlikely to change of its own volition. I've resigned myself simply to attempt to do what I can in the confines of this system, and to walk away, when I can, from the politics and craziness. I remember clearly the words of my preceptor who said, "Do one good thing for one person each day, and that is enough." I try to do that and hope that sometimes I succeed. I've been humbled enough to understand that just doing that is a tremendous task; just to avoid hurting people requires constant attention and thought. I try to be honest to patients and their families. I try to listen to their concerns and attend to them. I try to count to ten when I find my temper getting short. I try to walk away from situations when it becomes clear that I am not motivated to do what is in the patient's best interest. I no longer "turf" patients to avoid work, but because I think they'll get better care elsewhere. I avoid getting into ego battles with my peers and seniors. I try to listen to people who know more than I do, even if I hate their guts and consider them lousy doctors. I try to prevent my own ego from getting me into situations that I am not qualified to handle.

That I've completed my training and am now "board certified" in my chosen specialty has given me much more autonomy to achieve these goals. Credentials confer tremendous power in medicine, and people simply don't argue with me so much anymore. Plainly put, I am much freer to do things as I see fit now than I was as an intern or resident. Still, the system has rules I must obey, a number of which I don't agree with. I still follow the tenet of "cover your ass" no matter how much I disagree with doing what that necessitates. I still torture the hopelessly ill when asked or told to do so by their private physicians because I know refusing to do so would require quitting medicine altogether. Now, I merely torture these patients as gently as possible, and keep them as comfortable as they can be while I perform the *chu-cha*. Morphine, Demerol, and local anesthetic use rises dramatically whenever I am in the ER. I still perform procedures on patients that I consider cruel and inhuman if that is necessary to cover my own ass. The only difference now is that I get on the phone with the hospital's legal department beforehand to make sure I have to do it from a legal standpoint; the answer is inevitably yes. Sometimes I seek these situations out, egotistically assuming that I will be gentler and more humane to the patient and his family in performing such procedures than a number of my colleagues. I have been through the trial of catastrophic illness and death in a personal sense since I was an intern, and try to share my newfound empathy with the patient and family. Still, I remain hardened, and haven't yet been forced to skip lunch over a patient's or family's pain.

I've even eased up on my attitudes toward the docs that I consider "bad docs." I work on a salaried basis and write my own work schedule, which I consider a great luxury, and which frees me from any financial incentives in my work. Many of my peers have graduated to the exalted status of private attending, and the forces that prod them to attend their own financial and legal health at the cost of the patient's have become increasingly clear. Friends who started out wanting to help mankind are now faced with the need to earn six digits a year (before taxes) just to cover med school loans, mortgage, child care costs, and car payments. They do their best for their patients, but also have to keep a very close eye on the bottom line. I have been enraged when the doctors who have attended my own relatives refused to accept Medicare as payment in full for their services, but also understand that these payments often don't even cover costs.

Again, it is clear that money throws a wrench in the whole system, and those who are living off the fat of the shrinking health care buck are going to have to give up the game or we will all pay for their indulgences. This money is, after all, intended to pay for medical care and not making docs rich. I remain unforgivingly critical of high-powered specialists who tool around in Mercedeses and Jags, charging $250 for a fifteen-minute office visit and ten or twenty grand for five hours in the OR. This behavior, which clearly goes way beyond the concept of putting in one's dues and making a very decent living, has to stop.

I also try to remember internship every time I deal with a member of the housestaff. I felt robbed, cheated, and denigrated, and assume that most of the housestaff I work with today feel the same way. I try not to dump work on the interns I work with, and if I have to pull rank I attempt to do so without grinding anyone's face in it. I even toss out an occasional compliment, emphasizing recognition of the many jobs well done rather than the few done poorly. Miraculously, New York State has finally decided, after a million years of bowing to the AMA, to cut the hours of doctors in training. Now the maximum will be twenty-four at a stretch, eighty hours total a week, still slavery, but a vast improvement over the past. Big-cheese docs throughout the state have been in status epilepticus (constant seizures) since this announcement, much to my glee. I pray daily that the money for the added costs of this new system will come directly from the Mercedes and Jag crowd. I only regret that this book was not part of the impetus for the decision.

Finally, it remains clear to me that the vast majority of medical problems I see, my "bread and butter," remain primarily social, and not medical, in origin. Cigarettes, alcohol, and drugs; obesity; alienation; violence; and air, water, food, and land pollution remain by far and away the number one killers of Americans. Fix these problems and you'll see an end to the modern-day plagues of cancer and heart, pulmonary, gastrointestinal, and infectious disease. Raising the price of cigarettes to ten dollars a pack would do more for the health of the country as a whole than providing good medical care free of charge to all comers. Unfortunately, I went to medical school, rather than political activist school, and I guess I'll be staying in the Band-Aid business for quite a while to come.